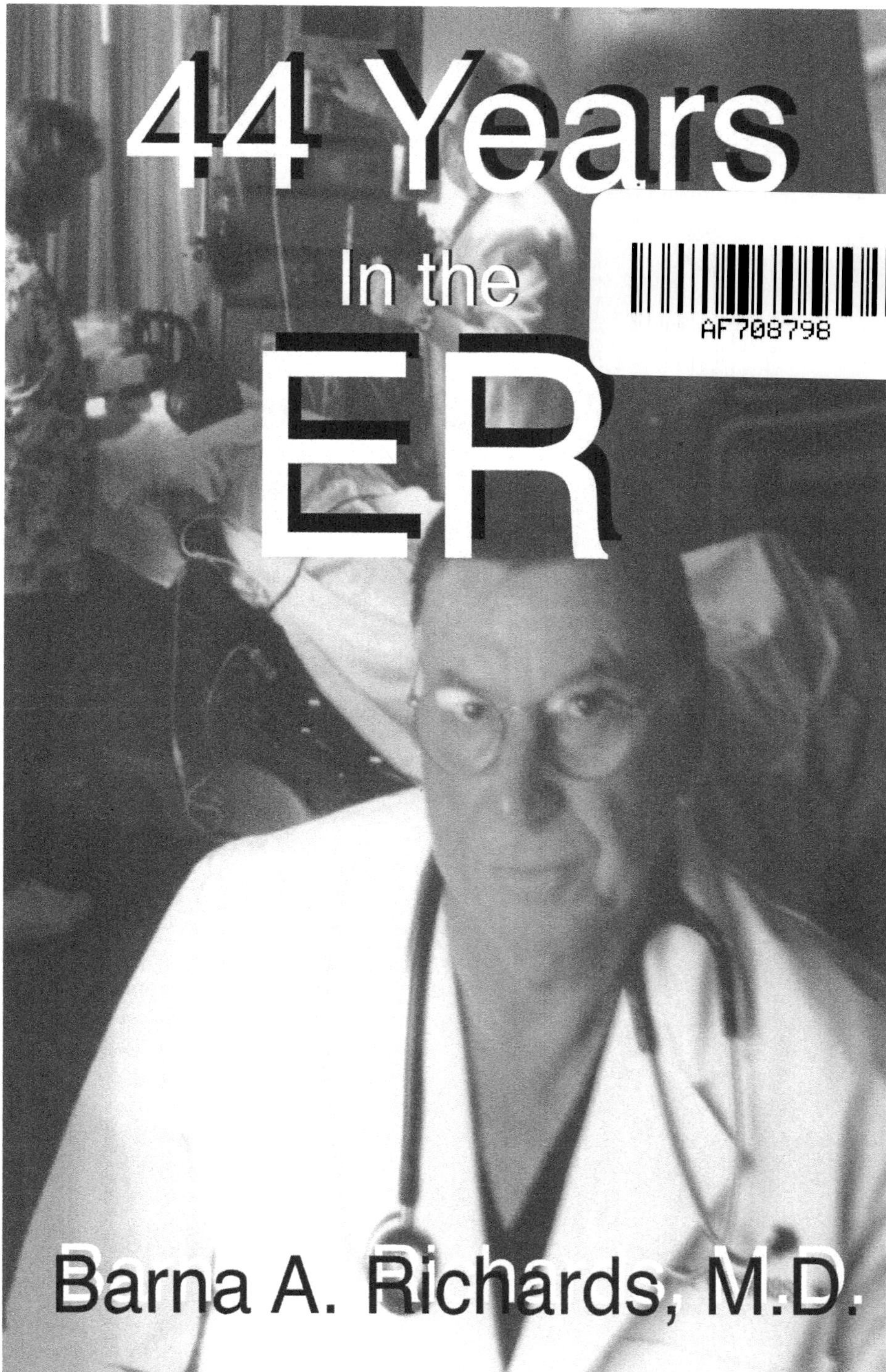
44 Years
In the
ER
Barna A. Richards, M.D.

Forty-Four Years in the ER

BY

BARNA A. RICHARDS, M. D.

ISBN-10: 1985233827
ISBN-13: 978-1985233829

The work of guest doctors were used with permission and belong to each author individually. Any comment made by contributing authors is not necessarily that of Barna Richards and he is not responsible for such comments. This non-fiction work is based on true events. However, the names of some people and/or places may have been changed to protect those involved.

Partner with SycamoreTreePress.com

Special Thanks to BCT Wordsmith

Dedication

I dedicate this book to all of those who have supported me in my quest to be a better emergency physician and leader of the emergency department. There have been many who have shared their knowledge and insight with me, and for whom I have great respect.

First are emergency nurses, who provide the majority of care in the ER. Their expertise is the essential glue that binds the physician's diagnosis and directions to a successful patient outcome. Without great nurses, neither the ER, the hospital, nor physicians could function in an effective manner. God love them, for there is a special place in heaven for them.

Next are the chaplains. One of the most difficult obligations of a physician is to inform a family that their loved one is critically ill or deceased. The chaplain rescues us and provides comfort and support to the family, as well as to the doctor. Their work is never done.

To my previous partners, both before and after emergency medicine became a specialty, and to all the ER doctors in all the towns, large and small, who are the safety net for our citizens, ill or injured, rich or poor, 24 hours a day, 7 days a week, 365 days a year.

To all the consultants who have responded to the ER, day and night for years, without receiving pay for their services in the majority of cases.

CONTENTS

Acknowledgments

My wife, Zotyne, who has tolerated my frustration over this book for the past year. Thank you!

Peggy Purser Freeman, editor/publisher, who has encouraged, cajoled, and gently pushed me to finish the book.

The Granbury Writers Bloc, who played a role in my decision to start this thing.

Introduction

Among doctors-in-training in 1963, the emergency room was commonly known as "The Pit." I never researched the derivation of the term, but it could be as in the bottomless pit. The doctor working a shift felt as if he's in a hole and will never ascend. Or the term may have come from pit as in pitiful. God knows, it can be pitiful. Most likely it came from pit viper because any doctor or nurse in the ER can get bitten by all sorts of creatures.

The doctor working the pit is known as the pit viper. He has to be pretty venomous for self-preservation. House doctors on staff in a teaching hospital pleaded with the pit viper to "be a wall," like a stone wall where no one gets past. Being a wall means the ER doc sends everyone home. If the patient needed admission, the intern had to do it. He may have had eight or ten admissions a night and be up twelve hours or more doing histories and physical exams, writing orders, doing procedures, and giving treatments. Then he had to call the resident who isn't very happy to leave the warm bed he's sharing with that cute little student nurse. Just kidding, I think. So the intern tells the emergency doc to "Be a wall."

Many a heroic story has been written about emergencies and emergency rooms. The stories in this book are true. Some will convince you that truth is stranger than fiction, funnier too—sometimes, and sad at other times. *44 Years in the ER* documents the evolution of the ER from the 1960s to the end of the century in the Dallas Fort Worth area—its history and its heroes.

Chapter 1
A Challenge of Mortality

In 1991, after 26 years in private practice, I gave up my security blanket—my practice—and traded it to become a full-time ER doctor. I was a dinosaur as an emergency physician. Most doctors my age had retired or slowed way the hell down. Only a semi-fool would quit a nice private practice to go into full-time emergency medicine, but I did, and of my own free will. No one ran me out of town, nor did the Board of Medical Examiners or my professional peers have any trouble with my skills. Some men climb mountains, race cars, or enjoy some other life-threatening endeavor. I chose emergency medicine to challenge my own mortality.

Looking back, my ER journey—filled with anxious nights, successful nights, and hellish nights of regrets—evolved with the history of the ER. That history documented change, progress and finally a specialty arm of medicine.

My ER experience began in the early 1960s at John Peter Smith Hospital (JPS) in Fort Worth, Texas. The emergency room at JPS consisted of an inadequate space for the number of walk-in patients and those from ambulances who flooded in each night. The small waiting room overflowed with very ill or injured patients, some had no place to sit. In some situations, the only resting place being the dirty floor, wreaking of contagion. The ambiance of the surroundings created a sense of decay and neglect, defeating the continuous effort of those who worked to keep it neat and clean. Vomitus, blood, debris, body odor, and the smell of dirty diapers, cigarette smoke and alcohol saturated the air.

Patients waited for hours, their moans and groans mixed with the cries of tired and hungry babies echoed and bounced against the walls. Sirens announced the arrival of victims of car wrecks, gunshots, domestic abuse, bar fights, and more.

Just inside the ambulance entry stood the triage desk, like a sentinel barring entry to the coveted treatment area. Everyone registered, waited and were sorted (triaged) to determine the severity of their emergency by a nurse and finally were seen by a young intern or resident who had already seen 25 to 30 patients.

In 1963, the pay for interns and residents was not a livable wage. Because of this, many of us "moonlighted" to bolster our income.

On one such evening, about ten p.m., while working in a small community hospital ER in north Fort Worth, a lady brought her child, a two-year-old girl, to the ER with the complaint of fever, congestion, and cough. These symptoms are responsible for a high percentage of visits to an ER and usually result in no serious consequences. However, a physician must always be aware of the possibility of the child with a fever and cough having something more problematic, such as pneumonia or, worse, meningitis. When I examined her I found that her temperature registered 104.4. Her face appeared flushed, pink, but she didn't appear dehydrated. She suffered from a mild otitis media (middle ear infection). The remainder of her exam seemed normal. Even though the lungs sounded clear, I ordered a chest X-ray and it was normal.

Children caused me the most concern because their condition can deteriorate quickly. I phoned the on-call doctor, related that I had a small child who might have meningitis, and asked, “Can you come and give a second opinion?” He said, “Oh, hell! Can’t you find something to treat the kid for and send her home?”

This left me with the obligation to do what I thought best. Obviously, he wasn’t coming and I wanted assurance that the mild ear infection caused her symptoms. Therefore, I decided I needed to do a lumbar puncture (spinal tap) to be sure she didn’t have meningitis. I doubt that a lumbar puncture had been done in that clinic in thirty years or so, and the assistant helping me had never helped to do one. The difficulty of holding a two-year-old still is like trying to subdue a wild animal. If she squirmed at the wrong time, the needle might not go to the correct location. The case could have a deadly outcome either way.

First, we located the equipment necessary to do the procedure. That took about thirty or forty-five minutes. All the while, the mother looked frightened and the terrified child cried. I felt frustrated and embarrassed that it took so long to get things done. I could have choked the on-call doctor for not coming to help me.

While I'm treating this child, my own life-drama unfolded about ten miles south in Fort Worth where my wife labored to deliver our first child at Harris Methodist Hospital. Of course, I missed the delivery. Fortunately, my wife’s mother had arrived a week earlier from west Texas to be with her daughter at her time of delivery.

Many more times in the next forty years, I would be

either late, called away, or absent for family occasions, but I chose this life, and I had to accept it.

My wife worked while I attended medical school. Now, as the sole source of income for our family, I worked all the time possible. With hospital bills, doctors' fees, and baby-needs, our expenses multiplied. Moonlighting became mandatory.

Some community hospitals required their medical staff to provide coverage of their ERs, and the doctors didn't want to take that responsibility. For that reason, the hospitals hired interns or residents to work nights, weekends, and holidays because we worked cheap and the regular staff physicians were relieved of the burden.

Concerned that a patient would come in and I couldn't adequately manage their care tormented me. There might be a person in a life-or-death situation where a more experienced doctor could save them and I might not have the ability to do so. Each time I heard an ambulance siren, I silently prayed that it would go someplace else. Even though I had been involved in treating some serious illnesses and accidents in the ER at JPS, I did have the benefit of experienced nurses and if I needed it, help from a resident. In this small clinic ER I didn't have that security.

But the patient in this case was a two-year-old. The fact that another doctor made a life-or-death decision for my wife and our first child in another hospital intensified my concern.

Meningitis constitutes a serious medical emergency. Children, or adults, can die in a short time if not diagnosed and treated within a few hours of the onset of symptoms, sometimes less. Knowing this, I struggled in a state of major agitation because of the delays. Getting an X-ray, trying to get the on-call doctor to help, finding the needed equipment, and instructing the assistant on how to hold the child, I did the procedure. To insert the needle into the spinal canal on a child who is frightened and struggling to get free of the restraint is like threading a needle with shaking hands in an ambulance on a bumpy road.

On the first attempt, my assistant couldn't keep the child immobilized enough. Understandably, she feared hurting the little girl. On the next attempt, we were successful. Elation soared through me as crystal clear spinal fluid dripped from the hub of the needle into the prepared vials. I sighed—clear fluid. Although it wasn't solid proof that the child had no meningitis, it encouraged me. If the fluid had been cloudy, that would indicate an increase of WBCs (white blood cells) and protein that results from infection in the spinal canal. Examined under the microscope, the fluid showed no WBCs. Convinced that she would be okay, I instructed the assistant to give an injection to treat the ear infection, gave mom some basic instruction on control of fever, to increase fluids, and to return the following day. The unhappy child pulled away from me, but mom looked relieved. I breathed easier feeling like an elephant of responsibility stepped off my chest.

***

In 1963, I served as an intern at John Peter Smith Hospital (JPS) in Fort Worth, Texas. Before 1979, a specialty in emergency medicine didn't exist. Those of us who were broke and hungry worked the emergency room to make ends meet. I moonlighted in the ER as an intern for minimum wage (about a dollar an hour). When I entered practice in 1965, I worked the ER to build my practice and make extra money.

Getting the hours in the hospital ER proved to be easy. However, getting paid for working was hit or miss, with minimal hospital funding for ER doctors, except what could be collected from patients, ended up spotty at best.

In my second year as a resident at JPS, a thirtyish year-old male arrived in the ER with a small wound to the chest, no blood pressure, no pulse, no respiratory effort, and he didn't respond to voice or physical stimuli. The heart monitor showed a complex of electrical activity.

Electrical activity without a pulse is known as PEA, or pulseless electrical activity, a very ominous sign. I picked up the chart and checked him right away. Seeing no immediate response, I considered the data. If dead, he hadn't been dead long. Even though we found no signs of life, he felt warm. The wound lay just to the right of midline—about one-fourth inch long. I couldn't harm him. He was technically dead. Pronouncing him dead and being done with it made logical sense and seemed the simplest thing to do. However, that little gremlin in the recesses of my brain told me, "No! Don't give up."

I decided to try resuscitation, but, how? The thought swirled in my head, and I knew time was the enemy. Time lost equals tissue lost, especially in the brain. I formulated a plan that seemed drastic, but he was dead. Anyway, you can't kill a dead man.

I followed that principle for the remainder of my career. I taught paramedics to do anything, even seemingly drastic deeds when a life is in the balance. *Besides, you can't kill a dead man.*

I asked the nurse to bring me a long spinal needle and syringe. I inserted it into the area just below the xiphoid (the little piece of cartilage at the bottom of the breastbone) and directed it toward the patient's heart. With no way to see where the needle tip needed to stop, I cautiously advanced the needle a couple of millimeters at a time.

I felt ambivalent about my trying to save him. Is this foolish? What if this case goes to review and I'm asked, "Why on earth did you waste time by sticking a needle in his heart when he was already dead?" I thought I could explain that. However, my doubts nagged me. What were the possibilities of success? Zero to none? The charge nurse stuck her head in the door and gave me a look that shouted, "What in the hell are you doing in there? We're busy out here."

That did nothing for my confidence. But I persisted and very slowly advanced the needle until blood came into the syringe. The needle tip could have been in the heart cavity, or a coronary artery, or the giant vein (vena cava) which wouldn't have helped, But as I withdrew blood, a pulse returned, weak at first, then stronger as I withdrew more blood. We called a heart surgeon and the operating room stood on alert. With his blood pressure at a reasonable level, we took him to the operating room.

I assisted the surgeon. When we opened the chest, we found a little blood in the chest cavity, a small tear in the pericardium (the sack around the heart) and a small hole in the right ventricle. We drained the blood from the blood-filled sack and put three sutures in the heart. We fixed the pericardial sack, closed the chest, and closed the incision.

In post-op, the patient did well, then went home five days later, and never realized that he had been snatched from the jaws of death.

His injury, called pericardial tamponade, involved the heart and pericardial sack. Blood fills the little sack around the heart and causes so much pressure that the heart can't expand normally, therefore it can't pump adequate amounts of blood to support circulation. As blood is removed from the space between the pericardium and the heart muscle, it decreases the pressure, allowing it to pump normally. The injury to the heart proved minimal

This remains, by far, the most dramatic "save" I've ever made. I admit that when the surgeon didn't give me a pat on the back or compliment my astuteness I felt disappointed. This case turned out to be a rare success story, accomplished by a young and relatively inexperienced doctor.

As this young and relatively inexperienced doctor, I could work the ER all I wanted in private hospitals because the more sane, private doctors wanted no part of the emergency room. Staffed by way of a call list, the entire medical staff worked on a rotation basis. Those who scheduled the ER considered anyone with an MD degree competent to treat emergencies. It may have been the philosophy of "any old port in a storm." A typical rotation included a pediatrician on Monday, a surgeon on Tuesday, a psychiatrist on Wednesday, an internist on Thursday, a general practitioner on Friday, an anesthesiologist on Saturday, an obstetrician on Sunday, etc., so on and so forth. You get the picture.

Most of these doctors neither felt competent nor did they desire to work the ER. The hospital required it. Can you imagine a psychiatrist treating your cardiac arrest? This is no insult to the psychiatrist. He wasn't trained to treat heart ailments. One can see the immense need for training in emergency medicine as a specialty. It was needed and eventually born with the development of Emergency Medicine specialty training programs. Prior to the institution of ER training, residency programs such as we experienced at JPS were the closest thing to ER training.

***

On another night at John Peter Smith Hospital, a twenty-five-year-old male walked into the ER with blood splattered over the front of his shirt. I rapidly raked through the hair on his chest looking for the wound but couldn't find anything but blood—no skin penetration. The man didn't say anything. A nurse came into the room and said, "What's that on his forehead? I examined his face and found a small wound just below the hairline. We finally got the story.

Earlier that evening, his wife came home to find him in bed with another woman. She put a 22-caliber pistol to his head and pulled the trigger.

I thought, *What's going on here?* He walked into the ER on his own strength. He didn't look like a man who had been shot in the head. When we looked at the X-rays, (CT or MRI scans didn't exist at that time) we saw the bullet lodged at the base of his skull. No skull fracture.

This had to have been one of the luckiest men in the world. The bullet penetrated the skin, traveled around the bone and stopped. It never entered the skull. After a short period of observation, and him with an industrial-strength headache, the hospital dismissed him. He won the lottery of life and didn't know it.

Please let me emphasize that doctors in the '50s and

'60s were well trained, competent, and, in numerous ways, more dedicated to hard work and the total care of their patients than many may be today. Emergency care proved to be a different matter because no training programs in emergency medicine existed. The ER operated as if no one needed to go to the hospital without an appointment. If they did have an emergency, the doctor available and his specialty brewed up potluck for patient care.

Later, after entering private practice, those of us who served as stalwarts of the ER worked double duty. We worked the office in the day and the ER at night. A typical scenario included going to the office in the morning, working until 5:00 that evening, go to the ER, work until 7:00 in the morning, travel back home to shower, and back to the office to work until 5:00 in the afternoon. After this full day of making rounds at the hospital, we got to go home, maybe to sleep, but more likely to answer phone calls part of the night.

We did these 36-hour shifts at least once per week, sometimes twice. I know that young doctors today look at me as I may have looked at my father when he said he walked to school barefooted, uphill both ways, to save his shoes for Sunday.

In the '60s, we weren't required to be present in the hospital at Arlington Memorial Hospital (AMH) but took calls from home. Not many people went to the ER for care then because almost everyone had a family doctor and would call him if they had a problem. The doctor managed most of the problems over the phone. As the old adage goes, take two aspirin and call me in the morning. If he couldn't solve the problem by phone, he got out of bed, many times dressed in suit and tie, and went to the ER to see his patient. You won't find many private doctors in the ER these days, except when one is on call for a given specialty. There are legitimate reasons for this; the private doctor probably doesn't feel comfortable in treating emergencies any longer, even though they are perfectly capable of managing the majority of problems which constitute most of what we see in the ER. Besides, it's inconvenient and his time is better spent in his office.

I can't say that things were perfect in those golden days either. Many times a patient waited hours for the doctor to finish dinner, a party, or whatever hanky-panky he may have been involved in before he decided to bless the suffering person with his presence in the ER. God knows not many doctors in those days knew as much emergency medicine as the well-trained ER specialists of today. Adrenalin, penicillin, and the surgeon's knife were the mainstays of emergency care and, on some occasions, penicillin may have sufficed, but surgery proved to be their choice.

In 1970, the powers that be decided it appropriate for a doctor to be physically present in the emergency room. We formed a group consisting of family doctors and surgeons to staff our ER. The family doctors became pretty adept at treating the majority of problems, and surgeons excelled at surgery, but I have recurring nightmares when I think of the average surgeon managing a child with meningococcal meningitis. Usually, he would call a pediatrician to manage the case. Surgeons were usually in charge of emergency rooms in teaching hospitals, presumably because only accidents were considered emergencies.

Surgeons in teaching hospitals did a great job of public relations back in the day. It seemed much more dramatic to have your life saved by surgery than by any other means. At least, so said public perception. Also, life-saving cardiac drugs and non-surgical procedures, considered commonplace now, didn't exist. All said and done, judged by the standards of the time, we did a pretty good job. Most ERs, many staffed by interns, experienced a similar history.

I can't imagine whoever thought an intern should be on the front lines of emergency care. Apparently, the CEOs watching the bottom line knew interns worked dirt cheap. In the '60s, when a patient needed admission to the hospital, the intern called another of his peers from the appropriate service to take over. If he needed help, he called a second-year resident and, if needed, a third-year resident could be called. Rarely did a staff physician come in at night. It's fortunate that the statute of limitations ran out or lawyers would have a heyday.

One night while on obstetrics (OB) during my internship, I had a lady who needed a C-section. I called the obstetrician on call and told him about the case. He said, "Why are you calling me?" I said that I thought he would want to come out to supervise the surgery. He said, "No! You and the second year guy can do it." I had never done a C-section, but the second year resident felt okay with it, and so I took the patient to the OR.

When I made the incision in the lower segment of the uterus, more blood than I had ever seen completely filled the wound, obscuring everything. *Oh, God! What have I done?* The resident reached in and pulled out the placenta, suctioned the blood, and everything became clear. There were no sonograms then, and the location of the placenta was unknown. My incision had cut into the placenta which bled like a stuck pig. I said a little thanks to God and the resident, without whom I might have had a heart attack. The mother and baby did fine.

Chapter 2
Pre-Hospital Panic

In the early 1970s, plus or minus a year or two, while on duty in the ER at AMH, the nurse called me to the phone. The call came from an ambulance attendant calling on a pay phone, his voice trembling with anxiety, speaking so fast that I couldn't understand him.

"Slow down. I can't understand you."

"Okay! Okay! Tell me what to do." The young attendant, probably a college kid, took deep breaths, huffing through the phone.

"What to do with what?" I snapped.

"What should I do with this dead man that we found here in the street."

"If you have a dead man, there isn't much to do. Call the police. Tell them you found a dead man in the street and they will take it from there."

"But we're not sure he's dead."

"Okay, tell me more about what's happening."

"We have a patient who is in a coma and we can't feel a pulse."

"Well, bring him in, and we'll see."

Minutes later, anxious and scared, sweat rolling down

their faces and wetting their shirts, they arrived and rolled the gurney into the ER hallway. The ambulance crew probably had never seen a dead person.

As they made the ninety-degree turn into the treatment area, they failed to slow the gurney. The man on the gurney sailed off onto the floor, landing with a thud. He lay motionless, no signs of life. I leaned over and checked his pulse. It beat strong and regular. I checked his pupils which looked equal and reactive.Then I quickly evaluated his skin—a little flushed but otherwise normal. No sign of trauma. No immediate life-threatening illness. However, he was very drunk, so much so that after sobering somewhat, he never remembered being so unceremoniously thrown off the gurney.

The ambulance attendants reacted with such nervous ineptitude over this seemingly serious situation that they failed to do the basic first aid to determine the life-revealing vital signs. We took X-rays of his head and neck and observed him for a few hours. The most serious problem to this hapless drunk consisted of a few bruises from the fall off the gurney. He woke with a bad hangover and went home to suffer. Today, we would have done a CT scan on his head and neck, but that technology wasn't available then.

Back in dinosaur times (before the 1980s), pre-hospital care consisted of ambulances furnished by the local funeral home and staffed by college students who liked driving fast and getting paid to do so. With little orientation to emergency care, other than a first aid course, they drove like a Mercedes on the Autobahn, scooped up the victim, and hauled ass. That personified pre-hospital treatment.

If you're curious as to why a funeral home would be so benevolent as to provide ambulance care to the city, the answer is economics. The first ambulance to the scene won the prize—the wounded or ill person. The concern for the welfare of the person came in second place. The prize was the non-survivor.

The funeral home got the bodies, thus the funeral and all the trappings, not to mention the headlines in the local newspaper sensationalizing the heroics of their attendants—the wild and crazy kid given a license to drive like a speed-demon. It became a toss-up as to whether the mad men in the ambulances killed more people than the usual traffic accident.

Our modern-day pre-hospital care offers sophisticated professionals, well-trained and fiercely dedicated paramedics. They work diligently, even though they are often under-appreciated and receive poor compensation for the wonderful work they do. I doubt they will ever get the recognition they deserve. As long as bureaucracies determine their worth, it's certain paramedics may never receive pay equal to their expertise.

I served as the medical director of EMS (Emergency Medical Care) for the cities of Arlington and Pantego, Texas, for the first ten years medical intensive care units existed in our city. Under my direction, we were among the first to allow paramedics to use their judgment to start an IV line and to defibrillate ventricular fibrillation (when the heart rhythm is just a quiver that doesn't pump blood to the tissues). Paramedics could also initiate drugs appropriate for the various emergent conditions. Other EMS systems in the area—Dallas, Fort Worth, and surrounding smaller cities—required the paramedics to get permission from medical control for all treatment. The ER staff usually provided instruction for all treatment. This delayed patient care when time was critical.

Working closely with the paramedics, I required extensive training in all of these procedures for paramedics in my units. They spent time in an ER learning to start IVs, and they helped me teach Advanced Cardiac Life Support.

I also taught them trauma principles, such as how to position pregnant women so the uterus didn't press on the aorta. In a woman in advanced pregnancy, the pressure of a large uterus can obstruct blood flow in the aorta, which carries blood to most of the body, if they are placed on their back. Therefore, they are placed on their left side.

Paramedics learned to check the ABCs (airway, breathing, and circulation) and trained to insert endotracheal tubes. They knew how to correct many deficiencies, as well as the basics of wound and burn care. The burn center at Southwestern Medical School in Dallas trained for burn wounds. Many of these procedures and principles were taught in their paramedic training, but I saw to it that these were reinforced regularly.

Because I worked closely with the paramedics and trusted their judgment, I gave them more leeway than other systems did. I don't know of any negative incidents that came from this liberal approach. However, the paramedics became more confident and proficient by being allowed to practice their skills. I only heard one comment from a fellow physician, who said, "I didn't know they could start IVs." He seemed okay with the change in using paramedics for procedures usually done by doctors or nurses. Of course, medics in the military were trained to do much more than the civilian paramedics, mostly because the military couldn't be sued.

Paramedic Shelley Lacy and her partner arrived at the scene of a major accident on the turnpike. They found a young man thrown from his vehicle who had suffered major injuries to most body parts and had no palpable pulse. With his chest crushed and his neck grossly swollen, he appeared dead by any practical judgment. However, he was young and the paramedics refused to give up when any chance of saving a life remained.

In poor light, in the middle of the highway, paramedic Lacy and her team inserted an endotracheal tube, put an intravenous line into a vein that could neither be felt nor seen. They started IV fluids. When the helicopter arrived, the patient showed a pulse and a measurable blood pressure.

In the hospital's surgery room, his opened chest revealed a severed aorta, just inches from its origin near the heart. Later, this man died in the trauma center with injuries that were incompatible with survival.

This incident occurred in 1993. These paramedics should have received commendations medals, the citizen of the year awards, but these wonderful people received a pat on the back from me and a few others who appreciated their work. It may have been different if the man had lived, but I doubt it. The patient didn't survive, but Shelly and her team gave him every chance possible.

The pleasure of working with many paramedics over my fifty years in medicine remains a fond memory and a source of pride in their accomplishments. They are not doctors, and the really good ones don't pretend to be. They work well with emergency physicians, who to a great extent, direct their actions. Rarely does controversy exist between them.

The pre-hospital workplace exists wherever a sick or injured person happened to be at that time. They respond to calls in the street, in homes with poor lighting, where family members might be hysterical, drunk, belligerent, and sometimes murderous. They do CPR, start IV fluids, defibrillate, intubate, bandage, splint, control bleeding, and then have to carry the patient out of the house over, around, and through furniture, kids, grandmothers, dogs, cats, drunks, and almost any other circumstance life might conjure. I have difficulty dealing with critical cases in the controlled milieu of the hospital. To function in the chaotic setting of a home beset by crisis becomes much more problematic.

War times developed a great deal of the pre-hospital care that is done today. Dominique-Jean Larrey, a French surgeon in Napoleon's army, developed "triage," a system of sorting out the various types of injury into categories based on which ones needed the most immediate care, in a descending order of four stages: most critical, urgent, less urgent, and deceased. They quickly discovered that the sooner they got the patient to a field hospital, the better the outcome.

Larrey's answer to the problem became known as the "flying ambulance." The invention of the modern day flying machines came after the Napoleonic wars, but Larrey's horse-drawn ambulances, coaxed to extreme speed for the time, soon owned the term "flying ambulance." Though he couldn't have imagined that ambulances would actually be flying one hundred and fifty years later, with the use of helicopters, recovery rates improved because of Larrey's prescience.

In successive wars – WWI, WWII, Korea, Vietnam, and the Gulf Wars – these principles progressively improved and helicopter transport helped to decrease the time to definitive treatment. We now call it the "golden hour," when getting an injured person to definitive care within one hour after the incident saves lives and limbs. Even better, the "platinum half-hour" became the next goal.

Chapter 3
An Unnecessary Death

One evening in 1964, while moonlighting at an area hospital, an event occurred that haunts me even today. Almost every doctor in town attended meetings in Dallas for the Texas Medical Association. I had covered the ER in this hospital enough that the doctors trusted me, and I felt pretty comfortable in my abilities at that time. Back then, emergency rooms in small hospitals rarely buzzed with activity and serious cases were unlikely. On this night, because I had a moderate amount of time in the ER in my training and rotations in surgery, internal medicine, and pediatrics, I could manage most any case.

A few hours into my shift, an ambulance brought a man in from a car accident. With normal blood pressure and no significant lacerations or obvious fractures, he complained of some pain in the left side of his lower rib cage, but the lungs were clear, with no obvious rib fractures. His abdominal exam seemed normal.

Fairly routine X-rays and blood tests for such an injury were accomplished and nothing stood out. I had some other patients needing care but checked on him periodically. I wasn't particularly worried about the accident victim at that time. Not too long afterward, he became agitated and said he felt like he was going to die. This most ominous sign got my attention. Actually, it scared me. Then he became pale and sweaty. His pulse rate registered 120. Short of breath, he complained of more pain in the left side.

The first sign of acute blood loss, or hypovolemia (low blood volume), is a rapid pulse. Unfortunately, a young healthy person may not develop these signs until a significant percentage, 30 percent or so, has been lost The nurse initially had been unable to start an IV, but this didn't seem important at that time. Now it did. She tried again and failed. I became more scared, actually, terrified is a better description. Without an IV, it was impossible to give fluids or blood. I knew I had to do something and started a cut down on the lower right leg. (a cut down is done by making an incision over a large vein so that an IV catheter can be inserted.)

I had done enough of these to know what I was doing, but it became more difficult to isolate a vein because the veins tend to collapse when there is inadequate volume to sustain their pressure. The patient again said, "I feel like I'm going to die."

My mind flooded with self-incrimination. I failed to get the cut-down completed before he arrested. His blood pressure hit zero, no pulse, unconscious, and blue. At that stage of shock, he had no real chance of survival.

We did chest compressions and mechanical breathing, but I knew it was futile at that point. He was dead. I wanted to die, too. A relatively young and healthy man had died under my care, and I felt completely to blame.

Maybe I hadn't paid as much attention to him as I

should have. I could have called one of the staff surgeons in to give me another opinion, regardless of his being in the meeting in Dallas.

As confident as I had been in my training, with all the approval I had gained from my mentors, I believed I was about as competent as anyone. Now, I suffered severe doubts. Maybe I'm not good enough to be in this profession in the first place, I thought.

Maybe I should consider quitting medicine altogether. Get a job that didn't put lives in my hands. However, I never had quit anything in my life,even when medical school seemed impossible in my first year, when several of my classmates quit. They, too, felt it was impossible. I stayed the course.

I never got over the guilt I felt because of this death, and it haunts me today—over fifty years later. I think of how it would have been if it had happened thirty years later when a CT scan would have been done and would have diagnosed a ruptured spleen or liver. He would have been taken to the OR and he would have lived. But we didn't have CT scans or many of the technological diagnostic choices then that we take for granted now.

Chapter 4
Bastard Orphaned ER

The emergency room used to be the bastard orphan of the hospital, and those of us in the business had difficulty accepting this. The ER is the entrée to the hospital. For many patients it's the first impression of the facility. Yet, CEOs, in the '60s, '70s and '80s denigrated the importance, cursed the "losses," and, at the same time, created cost-shifting accounting that rendered it impossible for the facility to show anything but red ink. Most businesses would cater to a department that has a volume of 41,000 persons per year (1990). Ironically, today those hospitals that don't have the high-volume emergency departments advertise for patients and make guarantees that the patient will be seen in 30 minutes or their visit will be free. Those who have it don't want it, and those who don't covet what they don't have.

The first community ERs I remember were one-room affairs. That's why they were called emergency "rooms." In 1988 our emergency department encompassed some five-thousand square feet and consisted of thirty-three treatment rooms, five offices, two break rooms, six restrooms, a conference room, and a waiting room that seated seventy-five or so. One could scarcely call that an emergency "room."

While still an intern, I felt scared to death all night

long, fearful that a true emergency would arrive. The real doctors were not very happy to be called in after they had worked all day.

Early in training I suffered diarrhea every time I heard an ambulance siren for fear that some disaster would appear and I wouldn't be up to the task. Fortunately, the disasters remained within the realm of my ability. I believe that fear of disaster is the reason I felt drawn to the emergency room. My thinking followed the path that if I could treat the immediate problem, I could always get a specialist to take over once the crisis ended.

Permit me a little pettiness here. The emergency doctor frequently isn't credited for the life-saving care. The attending physician comes in after the real emergency is over. He sees the patient for five or so days in the hospital, making rounds every day until the victim is discharged from the hospital, and the patient only remembers the attentiveness of the doctor who saw him/her the most. He tends to forget the one who saved his bacon.

During thirty years (1963 to 1993) of doing emergency care, there were numerous times when I was principally responsible for saving a life, always with the capable help of some very talented nurses, and never during that time did anyone come back to thank me or the nurses. I have wondered about this phenomenon many times. One tends to thank another for fixing a flat tire or opening a door for them, but not for saving their life?

In 1994, a middle-aged man walked into the ER complaining of chest pain. He sat on the gurney and immediately went into cardiac arrest. The nurse, Debbie, defibrillated him twice. He awakened with a very pained expression on his face, and said "Thanks, doc." He returned twice more to thank us. We greatly appreciated his words. Over the following years, two more individuals we had resuscitated returned to express their gratitude.

One of my good friends, a surgeon, had to come out about 3:00 a.m. one morning to operate on a lady who had come to the ER with a surgical condition. Knowing the surgeon had an early surgery scheduled the same morning, I apologized for having to call him out. He would get no sleep that night.

"That's okay, Barna," the doctor said. "The patient actually said 'thank you.' That's payment enough."

That touched me because the general opinion then, and remains today, that doctors are more concerned about money than caring for people. In this case, she had no means to pay, there would be no reimbursement.

Our society believes the greed-of-physicians myth. Between thirty and forty percent of our patients can't, or refuse, to pay for emergency care. We never know, nor do we ask if they can pay. Our hospital has never denied care to any individual for lack of ability to pay. I'm proud of that fact, even though if they all came in at once and paid for the entire free care we have given, we could retire in luxury.

In the early '60s, heart surgery wasn't a routine matter. They considered heart surgery experimental. Fortunately, I had experience as the fourth assistant on a patient who had a heart valve disease called mitral stenosis (the mitral valve is the opening from the left atrium to the left ventricle of the heart). The opening was too small to allow adequate blood to pass through.

As a junior student in 1962, a young lady patient assigned to me had such poor blood flow that she could only brush her hair one or two strokes at a time before she had to rest. She could walk about ten feet and required help to get back in bed. The day after her surgery, she could walk half the distance of the hall and could comb her hair without resting between strokes. I considered her surgery a miracle. She did, too.

Towards the end of my career, open heart surgery became much more routine—as long as I'm not the patient and the team isn't operating on me. Modern day heart surgery isn't anything to sneeze at. A doctor friend of mine sports a pig valve that replaced his damaged aortic valve. He's doing fine after thirteen years. Mechanical valves, heart transplants, and even the new regenerative procedures are much more successful than thirty years ago.

Like everyone else, some surgeons are weird, often with a strange sense of humor. The next case is a sample.

At Parkland Hospital, "The Lands" as doctors who trained in Parkland called it, the fourth-year surgery resident had a strange sense of humor. He asked questions—weird ones.

"Did you ever hesitate on the sidewalk?" He looked at the patient with a serious expression. "Did your mother ever give you a through of poultice?" He would say to the nurse "Give this man a shot of insulo-strepto-digicillin-mycin." Of course, there was no such drug. Fortunately, the nurses all knew he was a little different and paid no attention to his nonsense, because of his skill as a good surgeon.

This resident showed meticulous care of his postoperative patients. Following surgery, a person is likely to get atelectasis (kinda' the same as pneumonia) if they don't breathe deeply and cough up their secretions. It was considered bad form to allow your patient to develop atelectasis, and staff surgeons often chewed the asses off of residents who allowed it to happen. This resident removed a gall bladder on a man who was recalcitrant about coughing and he had to repeatedly chastise the man to get him to cough. When his exasperation had reached its zenith, he commanded in a loud, animated voice. "Cough, dammit, cough or I'm going to run this tube all the way into your lung and I bet you'll cough then." The man coughed . . . coughed hard, and his incision split wide open, intestines falling all over the bed. "Stop coughing! Stop coughing! Stop coughing, dammit!"

The patient didn't know what the hell had happened. He was finally just doing what the doctor told him to do, and now he was getting yelled at again.

Doctors in training tend to be a little strange anyway, with good reason. Stressed to the ultimate, they rarely sleep. On duty, they drink coffee constantly, and drink whiskey off duty, while trying to learn a lifetime (or six) of knowledge in a few years. All while cognizant that there is so much they don't know that it scares the hell out of them. It's fortunate that medical training involves so much overkill and repetition that even the average doctor is very well trained and competent. Doctors only become incompetent if they become alcoholics or drug addicts, or maybe conditions make them cynical for some reason or other, conditions such as contending with Medicare, HMOs, the IRS, frivolous lawsuits, or divorces.

Chapter 5
Sex in the ER

Frantically a young man ran into the ER screaming. "I'm bleeding to death." We calmed him down to get some sense out of his hysterical outcries. Blood covered the front of his pants, however, no other injury was apparent. When he lowered his pants, we saw a most amazing sight in living technicolor—a swollen, blue and bloody penis. A rubber band tied around the glans (head) effectively cut off the circulation. He reluctantly told the story. While having intercourse, he developed pain and noticed a great deal of blood. When he saw it was from his manhood, he panicked and tied the rubber band around it to stem the bleeding.

To maintain my professionalism, I left the room to laugh. A tear in the frenulum (a band of elastic tissue under the glans) of the penis caused the swollen organ to bleed like a stuck pig.

I called a urologist friend and told him the story. He fell out of bed laughing, couldn't go back to sleep, and came to the hospital to see this tumescent phenomenon. A few sutures fixed the problem and the patient was on his way, probably to be celibate for a while.

(First rule of controlling hemorrhage: put pressure on the bleeding site. Don't rub it. Don't put a tourniquet around it. Just put pressure on the bleeding. If it still bleeds, put more pressure on it. The bleeding will be controlled until you can get more expert care.)

Sex seems to play a larger role in society today than in more innocent times. There isn't necessarily more of it—people are just more open about it. The old ER days saw the ravages of promiscuity with boring frequency. Fifty percent of singles today are said to have chlamydia. Herpes was the great hysteria of the '80s. Venereal warts, trichomonas, and, of course, AIDS are all too common. Every ER doctor and gynecologist can recognize the PID shuffle (pelvic inflammatory disease, usually due to gonorrhea) at a glance. If PID isn't suspected in a sexually active female with abdominal pain, the doc made an error in judgment.

Bizarre sexual behavior also results in some unusual objects being found in strange places.

A rather embarrassed man came to the ER with a rectal problem. When I examined his orifice, I met with an obstruction close to the exit. He wasn't offering any information, so I looked with a speculum and found a green vegetable. Try as I might, I couldn't remove it. A surgeon was called, took him to the OR. He couldn't get a grip with the usual instruments, so he used a corkscrew, screwed it into the item and pulled out a large green cucumber just like the cork in a wine bottle. Before going to surgery, this humble vegetarian told me he had sat on a sack of groceries and the thing just popped in there. I believe it, don't you? Sure!

Almost anything imaginable has been removed from rear-ends and vaginas. Soap bars, light bulbs, gerbils, vibrators, wrenches, baseballs, bananas, apples, oranges, entire toolkits, and an array of fruits. I don't remember seeing a large watermelon—yet—but I won't be shocked when I do.

We should get hazardous duty pay for providing this professional service. One little needle stick while dealing with an AIDS patient can spell the end of life for the ER team. The hazards go with the profession. Early-day physicians had no protection from yellow fever, malaria, small pox, or any of the other plagues of their time, and yet they diligently plied their trade without whining. So I won't whine about our modern-day plagues either. I did fear contracting HIV from a patient's blood because I'm a rather dedicated heterosexual and would not enjoy the speculation my contemporaries might have if I came down with the disease.

A serious state of affairs exists from the sexual freedom in our society in the number of childhood pregnancies—children having children. These babies have little chance to become productive when their mentors are not much wiser than the baby itself. I don't have a solution, but a stronger family unit would be a boon. How do we accomplish that? I don't believe our benevolent government policies help either. Allowing food stamps, rent subsidies, medical care, and a rather freebee life style only makes it easier for these practices to be continued. Reality would be pretty discouraging to the prospective child-mother if she found none of those benefits available.

Hearing a sixteen-year-old patient describe that she was pregnant because she thought "a baby would be neat to play with" disturbed me. Of course, there was no money to pay for medical care or for the care of the baby. Guess who gets to pay for her new plaything? How about requiring them to work? Cleaning up some of the urban (and suburban) blight would be a good occupation since these children are not qualified to do anything but menial tasks, with a lot of supervision at that. Too cruel? I don't think so.

Sexuality is the most powerful urge in man's primal brain. As late as the 1960s I treated Vietnam veterans with everything short of nuclear fission trying to cure their very resistant form of gonorrhea. You might think the fear of AIDS would dampen the desire, or at least control it, but it ain't happenin'. The fear of disease starts just after the orgasm and goes away as soon as the next heat wave hits. This, too, isn't new to mankind. We just have to look back a few hundred years to realize that neither syphilis nor gonorrhea were curable, and some very notable characters were said to have died from these diseases, Al Capone and Adolph Hitler (not substantiated) for instance. Tertiary syphilis caused brain involvement, which rendered an individual deranged, or in some cases made them a vegetable for all practical purposes. Sex in the ER doesn't just involve patients. Doctors and nurses have been known to be participants also.

I slept in the interns' quarters in the wee hours when a banging on the wall of the next room awakened me. In my half-asleep state, I assumed someone was trying to wake me up. I went to the door, but no one was there. I returned to bed and the noise continued. I knocked on the door of the offending room and a nude doc opened it, sweaty and disheveled. When a little female voice said, "Come back to bed, baby," the mystery was solved, but I didn't sleep much that night.

One of my contemporaries of the time, a Clintonesque character, was thought to have spent more time in the back seat of cars and no-tell-motels than in the hospital. The favorite target of nurses, this guy couldn't help himself. Not that he wanted to. One night when he went out foraging, I asked him to bring me a pizza. Winter raged in full force, and when he returned with the pizza, it was almost frozen. He wasn't. He'd been hard at work at his favorite pastime for three hours or so while my pizza lay in the frigid environs of the automobile seat.

Interns and student nurses make a very volatile mix. The romance of saving lives and working in close proximity, at an age when hormones are out of control and idealism is in full bloom, create an environment for many romantic interludes and some shotgun marriages that don't always work out. A doctor who is married at the beginning of his internship may not be in the same state of marital bliss at the end of the year. He is a target, and there are many arrows aimed at the appropriate anatomy.

Nurses at a small community hospital were commonly known to visit the doctors' quarters for a quickie in the early morning hours. A surgeon acquaintance from England said that he always felt slighted if he didn't have a student nurse to warm his bed when on call.

God should have made an on and off button for sexual instincts. "On" for procreation and "Off" the rest of the time. That would save at least half the misery of mankind. Some genius would figure how to short-circuit the system, though, probably a computer nerd.

Chapter 6
What is an Emergency Doctor Anyway?

Until 1978, emergency doctors were considered a strange lot. Some say we still are. They consisted of interns or other doctors in training, part-timers who had private practices, such as myself at the time, and a few full-timers who didn't want the responsibilities of private practice. Needless to say, the quality of care varied greatly. That care depended on the interest of the doctor on duty in Emergency Medicine (EM) because no definite guidelines existed. Since surgeons had been in charge of emergency rooms in teaching hospitals for eons, they jealously guarded their turf, not wanting to relinquish their hold on that area of medicine.

In many institutions, mostly teaching institutions, in the 1980s, their recalcitrance has slowed the development of emergency medicine training. In the late 1970s, residency programs were developed in EM, and the American Board of Medical Specialties recognized the specialty in 1979.

By 2009 EM had become one of the most sought after training programs in the U.S. by doctors deciding on a specialty. For a few years, since there were insufficient numbers of doctors in this area, those of us who were not trained specifically in EM, but definitely experienced, were allowed to study for, and take, the exams for specialty certification. This is what I did in

1988. We all took the same tests, no favoritism or "grandfathering" in the program.

An emergency medicine resident works four years after medical school to complete his training. The training includes emergency care in every conceivable area of medicine with great emphasis on the most immediate, life-threatening conditions, such as cardiac arrest, serious trauma, infectious diseases, pediatrics, OB-GYN, and surgical emergencies. We don't do the majority of surgery but manage the diagnosis and contiguous care until the surgeon takes over. We do suturing, splinting of fractures, and other procedures that can be done in the setting of the ER. Some of the brightest minds in medicine now practice the specialty, and in most urban hospitals, one can feel comfortable he/she is getting the best of care in the ER.

Emergency doctors do more teaching than the average physician. I believe this stems from the fact that we work closely with paramedics and nurses. This requires a team effort to be more efficient. One must be prepared in order to teach. Therefore, a lot of time is required in preparation. Advanced Cardiac Life Support, trauma courses, pediatric life support, as well as many less formal seminars and teaching sessions, are courses the doctors take and teach to others.

Most medicine specialties are subject to horrible hours, but few are constantly required to staff their area of responsibility 24 hours a day. The shift work is a major cause of doctors dropping out of the specialty. One works days, evenings, nights, weekends, and holidays. The circadian rhythm becomes destroyed. The brain and body don't know when to sleep. When fatigue becomes overwhelming one may sleep fourteen or so hours and awaken to find that it's only 3:00 a.m. Now, he can't go back to sleep and has to be at work at 7:00 a.m. He goes to work tired as hell and the vicious cycle starts all over again.

When he finishes his shift, sleep may come or it may not. If it does, it may be three hours or twenty-four. You never know, but it's certain that a day off isn't a day off when you've been up all night. Ravaged by memories of the multitude of problems faced under the most difficult of circumstances, it's difficult to turn the brain off until the sleep center in the old brain says, "Wait a minute, I've had enough of this crap. I'm going to sleep. You can do whatever you want to, Body," My brain screamed, "but mission control is outa' here."

Chapter 7
The Anatomy of a Doctor

To be a doctor was the ultimate goal for me. Because of my humble beginnings and my high regard for doctors, it never entered my thinking that I might achieve that lofty position. It seems ironic that I didn't consider the possibility until after I had flunked out of college the first semester—not an auspicious start. As a physician, I have difficulty overcoming my humility in order to adequately describe the unique attributes that are required to achieve an MD degree and the title of "Doctor of Medicine."

There are many individuals who have the innate intelligence to make the grades required to go through pre-med and medical school. Along with ability one must have stamina, persistence, and humility in order to accomplish the goal. A young person sets out "to be a doctor" not fully understanding what that entails. In any college freshman class, there may be several hundred who are pre-med majors. It sounds good to the girlfriend or the boyfriend, and there are many who claim that dubious title, but as time passes, the numbers diminish very rapidly, not because of lack of ability, but mostly a lack of commitment. I had one acquaintance who ranked as close to genius status as I can imagine. He attended medical school because his mother wanted him to be a doctor. He easily made the grades for pre-med, but had little interest in medicine and flunked out the first year. College pre-med courses are not average and are difficult, whether one attends Harvard or any university.

The social life suffers. Not all pre-med students are bookworms who prefer a book to a party, but the commitment to the goal has to overcome the natural urge to take the fun road. That "No Fun" road was difficult for me because I loved the social life, booze, girls, fishing, and hunting. I had to give up almost all of that. I didn't have the money to be a playboy anyway. The solitude of study weighs heavily when there is beer to be drunk and girls' company to be enjoyed. Eyes ache and the head throbs from looking through a microscope for hours at a time. The stacks in the library catacombs aren't a place for great social intercourse, but they are a sanctuary for one who knows he is vulnerable to the temptations of life. He escapes there to avoid the distractions that would surely occur if he allowed natural instincts to prevail. These are sacrifices. Not everyone understands what the word means, but most successful people in any field of endeavor have made many sacrifices.

For the remainder of one's life, the devotion to duty as a physician continues. No excuses accepted. Perfection may not be achieved, but it's expected, and failure is met with ignominy, as well as disapproval by the patient and family, not to mention a possible lawsuit. Personal life is often secondary and suffers. Financial security is only considered later in life when it may be too late to make it a reality. Being a doctor is its own reward during our productive years, and when we wake up to the realization that no one, other than those whose lives we have touched, really cares, it's too late. We can't go back and say "Wait a minute!" I worked hard, did it gladly, and was pleased I could. Unfortunately, I destroyed my personal life for my career in medicine and didn't achieve great wealth.

These are long days, weeks, months, and years of commitment, not a few months, or a few years, but a lifetime. What is a night of interrupted sleep to a person? Many years of it has its effect on body and mind. But it's worth the sacrifice as long as there is some appreciation—a "thank you" from a person in need or the words of a child who says, "That's my doctor."

I played in a charity golf tournament once, where celebrity athletes and entertainers were among the participants. Children scurried around the course and collected autographs from players from the Dallas Cowboys, Texas Rangers, country and western singers, and individuals of the local media.

A young boy came up to my golf cart and said, "Can I have your autograph?"

I very honestly said, "Son, you don't want my autograph, I'm nobody." He said "Yes, you are. You're my doctor." I was very flattered—it almost brought me to tears. I signed his program, doing my best to make it legible. In spite of my golf game, his gesture made my day a complete success.

Chapter 8
The Damnedest Reasons

"Go to the ER," the lawyer says, caring not that they can't pay. *I have a cure for the great debt national, avoid ER for things irrational.~B.A.R. 1997***.**

Neither rhyme nor reason can explain the strange things that bring a person to the ER. A common question often asked of a patient is "What brings you to the ER tonight, Mr. Doe?" Mr. Doe responds, "A taxi." "Oh! Okay. Thank you."

A young, wimpy kinda' guy complained of a fish bone in his finger. The story was that he was eating in a restaurant and stuck himself with a bone. I looked at his finger and couldn't see anything. He insisted. "It's right there!" I still couldn't see anything. I asked the nurse to bring me the magnifying glass because this man was serious about this wound. He was immediately offended that I was unable to see the result of his assault by the microscopic "Jaws" and I assumed he would sue me for failure to diagnose along with the restaurant's failure to restrain their attack perch.

Aches, pains, bumps, and strains,

Little rashes and minor smashes,

Backaches for months and fevers anew,

Not several, but quite a few.

During a particularly bad ice storm one winter day, a lady came to the ER for back pain. I asked her when it started and was it a lot worse today. She responded that it had been the same for years and was not really changed. When I inquired why she decided to come on a day when she might have a car wreck or a fall on the ice, she said "I just got tired of it." In my somewhat logical mind, it seemed rather strange for one to chance serious injury for a condition that was chronic and no different from previous years.

I have always found it humorous that no one ever "goes" to the ER. They are always "rushed" to the ER, no matter if their complaint is a toothache, mosquito bite, or heart attack. Not so humorous are those who call 911 for non-emergent conditions such as a sprained ankle. On many occasions, they just want a ride to the hospital.

Daddies are particularly hysterical when their little girl gets a boo-boo. Baby girl needs a plastic surgeon for a cat scratch. That's a mega-buck abrasion on a good day. In my private practice, I encouraged patients to call me with their midnight complaints, and many emergency visits were avoided. It isn't necessary to take the child with a fever to the ER at the first blip of the thermometer over 98.6. Neither is a sprained ankle a life-threatening event, nor an asymptomatic rash, nor a cold, nor a hell of a lot of other office-visit types of problems. The HMOs have created the very monster that their multi-million-dollar-per-year CEOs wish to avoid. By destroying the doctor-patient relationship, people don't have the comfort of calling their family doctor to get reassurance, and the doctor who does not know many of his patients because they have to change doctors every time a company finds a cheaper deal, feels threatened of a lawsuit if the patient is given any phone advice that may not be absolutely correct, says "Go to the ER."

The so-called "managed care" has created a logjam in doctors' offices because those who have pre-paid care with a minimal co-pay feel free to go to the doctor for minor problems. They would never consider going if they had to pay a reasonable fee for the same service. Free service, or pre-paid service, results in a loss of common sense, which is much more likely to prevail when one has to consider if the service is worth the cost. Of course, this "ain't politically correct," but I have confidence that neither big insurance nor big government is going to be very successful at achieving accessible medical care in a timely manner. A doctor and patient who have mutual trust and liking for each other results in less testing, fewer visits, and lower ultimate costs. The doctor's office logjam results in more emergency visits because the doc just can't see everyone who wants to come into his office. This means the person with a problem goes to the always-available place—the ER, the very place the HMOs hate the most but is also the facility that bails their clients out frequently.

Everyone in a car wreck MUST go to the ER, even if they have no pain, no cuts, no nuthin'. If anyone doesn't think attorneys raise the cost of medical care, just calculate the number of needless, absolutely silly, emergency visits caused by the common belief that one must be examined immediately after an accident. Insurance companies share the responsibility also. Of course, the physician is a problem, too. He orders too many X-rays. Why? It's the attorney thing, stupid! If a witty bitty fracture is missed, heah' cum de' judge.

Conservatively speaking, billions of dollars are spent on really stupid visits to the ER for legal reasons.

Please don't sue me for discouraging a visit to the ER for a legitimate reason. I'm speaking of STUPID VISITS. Only the patient can determine his/her definition of an emergency. I can't do it sitting at this computer, but some common sense would tell one that a routine sprain or chigger bite isn't a life-threatening emergency, Did I say "common sense?"

There is an upside to unnecessary ER visits; it allows us enough volume to afford to pay highly qualified doctors to staff our ERs, and we, as a profession, must come up with a method of maintaining a reasonable income, charging reasonable fees, or else we will be back to the days of part-timers not so qualified to treat the real emergencies.

Chapter 9
Drug Seekers in the ER

The Hippocratic Oath urges physicians to relieve suffering, always. Many times that is all we can do and drug seekers have taken full advantage of this benevolence. The Drug Enforcement Administration (DEA) disdains the frivolous prescribing of narcotics and they have been known to entrap unsuspecting doctors by sending a shill with a feigned ache or pain to a physician. If they decide the doctor wasn't discriminatory in his prescribing, he may find himself facing charges. Most of us don't live in constant fear of the DEA because they usually reserve their energies for the real offenders, but it's a concern.

Migraine sufferers have a difficult time getting needed treatment because emergency nurses and doctors have an ingrained suspicion of them, assuming they are abusers. This is a terrible disservice to the true migraine patient whose pain is excruciating. They're often placed on the bottom of the priority list and may wait much too long for treatment.

My philosophy is to give anyone with apparent severe pain the benefit of the doubt, preferring to give a fix to the junkie than to deny pain relief to the real sufferer. Don't confuse me with "Doctor Feel-Good," I get very upset with abusers, as some of the following tales will describe.

A mother-daughter tandem was in adjacent stalls in the ER. I encountered Mama first and learned that her chronic back pain had just become acute. She couldn't possibly wait to see her neurosurgeon for her pain medicine, which happened to be two drugs, both of which are highly addictive and are just loved by junkies. My antenna was up. I saw the daughter and, guess what, she needed the same drugs. My periscope went up higher. I gave them both something benign and dismissed the incident as another routine event in a day's work. They had just vacated the premises when the nurse called me. "Doctor, look!" Foolish me. I looked. There on the floor of the treatment room was a very sizable pile of feces. We have heard of people being "pissed off," but this was much more solid matter. We named her "the woman who crapped out."

One of those long-haired guys, disheveled and unwashed, wanted his favorite pill, a really infamous junkie drug, called Percodan. He was such an obvious drug seeker that he couldn't have fooled a fool. I refused his drug but gave him some reasonable prescription instead. When he left the ER he passed me as I sat working on a chart in the nurses' station. He shot me the bird, wadded the prescription up, threw it at me, and said, "You can stick this puny crap up your ass!" Well, I didn't, and he really was angry when I laughed at him. I wondered why my tire was slashed when I left work that night. Probably just coincidence.

Another hopeful seeker presented to me with a heart-rending limp, racked with such pain that he dramatically crashed to the floor, being very careful not to hurt himself in the fall. He loudly demanded, "Give me some ##**# pain medicine." I did him the courtesy of an examination, which also caused much dramatization and expletives, after which I offered him crutches and a mild pain prescription. He cursed me and the nurses, threatened that I would be hearing from his attorney (court-appointed, I'm sure), and with a woeful struggle made for the door. I happened to go out on the ambulance dock to talk with some paramedics when, lo and behold, our pitiful cripple ran to the waiting car of his accomplice like an Olympic sprinter, jumped into the front seat and sped off…probably to the nearest ER for another attempt. From the way he sprinted to the car, I wondered if I had cured him just by laying on of hands. Think so?

A young woman who had been a private patient of mine in years past frequently came to the ER "needing" a cough medicine with codeine. I didn't remember her being hooked on the drug, but she obviously loved it. In my earlier private practice, I felt compelled to monitor patients to be sure they weren't abusing drugs, but this one must have slipped through the system, or she developed the habit after I left my practice for the ER. Whatever the reason, she became a nuisance to the ER staff and physicians and we, as diplomatically as possible, told her that she could no longer receive a prescription for her cough medicine in the ER and would need to get her future medications from her personal physician.

The real slick drug abusers who used the ER as their "dealer" developed a lot of expertise and cool tricks. For example, they could mimic a kidney stone by screaming, as with agonizing pain, gagging with feigned vomiting and holding their back on one side or the other. The nurses and doctors were pleased when the guy forgot which side he had indicated as the locus of pain and sometimes changed sides. He would then bite his cheek, or prick his finger, bringing blood that he would surreptitiously try to introduce into his urine to substantiate his claim. He would become upset when we sent a male (or female, as the case might have been) staff member into the restroom with him to be sure he wasn't adding his "proof" to the specimen. These guys usually were not successful in their game of chicanery, but they were persistent and might try several different ERs in one day, looking for a less vigilant doctor.

Another common ploy was "I'm out of town and forgot my Oxycontin prescription."

"Sure you did," I said to myself. In my rejoinder to this person I sometimes would say, "Well, let me call your doctor and get his approval," knowing well that I wasn't about to give this faker a narcotic prescription.

"Oh my, he's out of town." They often answered.

To myself I'd say, "Well, I guess you are SOL." To the patient, I responded, "I'm so sorry. I just can't give you a narcotic prescription." Wasn't going to anyway.

Drug addicts are a sad lot of humanity, but the saddest are those who overdose and either succumb to the drug or act in such a way as to be dangerous to themselves or others. Rodney King comes to mind. But he got rich from his deranged aggressive behavior, thanks to some overzealous Los Angeles cops. Our ER experienced a similar patient on the same drug, phencyclidine, or PCP. This man became uncontrollable as he attacked the nurses and other staff while being evaluated. Not knowing the reason for his behavior, tests were attempted to be done, and he wouldn't allow anyone to touch him. Somehow, he was taken to X-Ray, and, while in the X-Ray department, he attacked the tech. Two cops happened to be in the ER and went to help. The patient began to throw people around like rag dolls, including cops. When I entered the fray, there were two cops, two male techs, and two nurses desperately attempting to control him. Suddenly, he went limp. He died, much to the dismay of everyone involved. I never heard of any consequences from this case.

Chapter 10
Two Strange Cop Stories

A police officer sat on the gurney in no great distress.

"My tooth hurts," he said. On further questioning, it was revealed that he had been shot in the back of the head. The bullet went through the head and exited through the mouth, breaking the tooth. He had no apparent neurological deficit, was fully awake, moving all extremities, and completely lucid. A CT scan revealed a trail through the brain but no major brain injury. A neurosurgeon was consulted, the man was observed for a while and dismissed with no permanent damage. This toothache will be, forever, the strangest one I will ever see.

An ambulance delivered a policeman who had been shot in the head to the ER. One would expect the officer to be moribund, or at least comatose or paralyzed. He was neither. In fact, he sat upright on the gurney and only complained of a tooth ache as I entered the treatment room. He didn't mention pain in the head, dizziness, weakness of either extremity, difficulty walking or speech. The neurological exam revealed no deficit. A CT scan did show some trauma but no intracranial bleed. The only abnormality on his exam was an incisor tooth broken in half. I consulted a neurosurgeon who admitted the patient to the hospital but released him in24 hours with no apparent permanent disability.

Now, those who are skeptical of the veracity of this story may join me in my disbelief. This happened over twenty five years ago, and I sometimes wonder if I dreamed it, but then, I did experience this incident and felt confounded and dismayed as it played out. There is no way to explain how this happened. This will remain the strangest toothache I have ever seen.

A female police officer came to the ER with a gunshot to the lower leg, accompanied by her partner who related the story as follows: "We were finished with our shift, and we usually unload our firearm at that time. As my partner jacked the shells from her 9mm Glock, the unfired shell hit the concrete and exploded, and the bullet hit her in the leg." I reflected on this, since I have unloaded many guns; rifles, shotguns, and pistols, and I never have had something like that happen. Her partner then said "this isn't the first time she did this. It happened to her once before, also." I think the odds of this occurring to one person on two different occasions is like being struck by lightning twice, the odds of which are 1 in 9 million. Her experience made me much more cautious when unloading a gun, and I always found a soft landing area for the unspent shell.

Chapter 11
Nurses in the ER

Emergency nurses, like emergency doctors, are a different breed, or maybe they are born masochist. Willingly, they jump into tumultuous and catastrophic situations, and their deranged brains seem to thrive on the chaos of the untidy maelstrom. Their reward—a patient saved from the jaws of death. The mess can be cleaned up later, after which they wait for the next disaster that may help to attenuate their vast adrenaline pool.

A good nurse is a great asset in any part of the medical milieu. In this treatise, I'm speaking of ER nurses in particular, and I have had the honor and privilege to have worked with many excellent ones. Not all emergency nurses are specially trained by the certification board (CEN). The certification has been available since 1980 but wasn't recognized by the American Board of Specialty Nursing until 2007. Similarly, board certification for emergency doctors wasn't made possible until 1979. The lack of certification doesn't imply that they were not competent, but certification affirmed that they had completed a course of study, passed the test, and complied with certain standards. Having recently spoken with one of my nurse friends who is certified, he tells me that the majority of ER nurses aren't certified, but hospitals are now highly recommending they do so.

Whether certified or not, the nurses I worked with over forty-four years were excellent, for the most part. I recall a number of times that their knowledge, experience, and ability to recognize a patient who needed immediate care saved many lives. The triage (sorting out) nurses, who immediately encounter the patients, are critically important to recognize and separate the real emergencies from the “can wait” ones. This can be the difference between life and death, for to fail to take the acute MI (heart attack) patient to the major treatment area in a timely manner can result in a cardiac arrest in the waiting room—a definite faux pas, not to mention a dead patient. Next in importance are the nurses in the major areas. They are well-versed in the medications and procedures needed for potentially fatal cardiac rhythms, and they usually have the appropriate drugs prepared and ready before the doctor orders them. That was my experience on many occasions, and it comforted me to have their expertise so readily available.

Fifty-Year-Old Overweight Female with a Nonspecific Complaints

The lady didn’t seem terribly ill. She was a fifty-year-old female, overweight, and had several nonspecific complaints, including shortness of breath. She had been dismissed from our hospital a few days earlier but had gotten progressively worse over that time.

The emergency doctor had done an extensive history and physical exam and found no definitive cause for her symptoms. While he was speaking with her attending physician, the lady became hysterical and began to hyperventilate. Two nurses were at her side and called the doctor to see her. Immediately thereafter she went into respiratory arrest. She was very rapidly intubated, and all life support measures were quickly instituted. While being ventilated (breathing for her), she was taken to the major medical area where further care could be given. In spite of being adequately aerated (providing oxygen and mechanical breathing), her face and neck were plethoric (purple). Her pulse rate became more rapid, and the blood pressure was dropping. This person was dying, and the cause was not apparent. An external pacemaker was put into place to stimulate heart contraction, and an echocardiogram was done to detect heart activity. She never responded to any of these interventions and expired.

The nurses were despondent. They had given care to her for over three hours and felt sickened that the outcome was death. A large part of their life seems to go every time a disaster like this occurs, and one wonders how many parts they have to give.

The nurse and doctor, heart heavy and remorseful, resignedly go to the family room where the anxious husband and children are waiting, their faces showing both fear and hope at once. The terrible truth is told. Disbelief. Cries of Why? Why? Why her? “She was alive just an hour ago! Couldn’t you have done something to save her life? My God, I don’t believe she’s dead.” The doctor and nurse feel something they never knew they would have to experience. It’s a depression that is total hopelessness and despair mixed with the guilt that arises from failure to save a life. Even knowing that this life couldn’t be saved, except by God, the remorse remains.

If you, dear reader, ever question why a doctor or

nurse seems to be cold and uncaring, try to get into their brain and look at the memories of twisted bodies, of abused children shaken to death by an irate boyfriend, teenagers with the back of their head blown off and brains and blood staining the back of their shirt, of people dying in front of your very eyes in spite of all you know, or anyone knows. Consider the "what if's" and "should I have's" and all the sleepless nights, questioning if anything more could have been done. Could someone else have done better? Should I be in this profession? Maybe I should quit. Perhaps I'm not good enough. God, I'm a lousy person.

Alarm clock rings, lousy person showers, gets dressed, goes to the hospital, takes a lot of deep breaths, pulls the shoulders back like daddy told us to do, looks the security guard in the eye and says " I'm doing fine. How are you," says same to the staff, gets into the battle, and it all starts over again. Maybe it'll be a better day…and maybe worse. The only means by which those of us who deal with death and destruction of human flesh can continue to perform in a competent manner is to push into the recesses of the brain those horrible events and move on to the next person in need of our expertise.

In the West Texas oil fields when things were not going well, an old tool pusher used to say "We have a good crew, but this well is a sombitch. Sometimes it goes on like this for days, then it gets worse." He was making a statement about life that I have found to be very true.

The family wanders out of the hospital. Tears and hugs. Hugs and tears. Disbelief prevails in spite of full knowledge of the truth. Uncertain faces. *What do we do? Mama is gone, wife is no longer with us. How will we survive?*

The emotional exertion from fear and uncertainty and the burden of grief fall on them as they shuffle in a stupor and seek their various means of transportation to go to a mutual grieving place.

It's not been a good day!

Chapter 12

Malpractice Threat as it Affects the Emergency Doctor

The ER physician is very vulnerable to lawsuits. The milieu is one of chaos and uncertainty, compounded by large volumes of patients, neither of whose numbers or timing can be controlled. Every patient must be evaluated in a timely manner. Long waiting times are inevitable, and those in the waiting room are of particular concern. Rapid triage has helped, but some with serious problems can be overlooked. Even when management of the case met all standards, there are those who die or have a bad outcome. The best of care, provided by the best of physicians, can result in a bad outcome and a suit might be filed. Desperate attorneys file questionable, or wrongful, suits. These make me furious.

I have no real argument with a lawsuit when care failed to be adequate or egregiously wrong, but frivolous lawsuits are a travesty, serve no good purpose, and can be devastating to the one who is wrongly sued. I fell victim to three lawsuits, and only one had any merit. The others never should have been filed and were dismissed. In one case, it became obvious that the attorney never read the case before filing the tort. I think this attorney deserved to be sanctioned by the bar, but lots of luck on that happening. Do the threats of litigation cause increased costs of medical care? I believe so, but if a doctor is concerned that something might be missed by not doing a particular test, perhaps he should have done that test, regardless of the fear of lawsuits.

Litigation is rife in our society, certainly not limited to medical issues, and has come to be a way of life. The fact is, that in the U.S. there are too many lawyers, some of whom will sue anyone, anytime, for any reason, but that isn't an indictment of the profession as a whole.

Chapter 13
Some Doctors I Have Known and Some Stories They Tell

Contrary to popular belief, physicians are not cut out of a mold, nor are they cloned as might be futuristic humanoids. They come from all parts of the world and from many diverse cultural and economic backgrounds. It's impressive to me that a son or daughter of wealth makes the sacrifices to become a physician. It may be more understandable that a person of humble beginnings has the drive and commitment to attain the MD degree. Obviously, the person of lesser means might be expected to have more incentive to achieve than the one whose financial life is already secured. In either case, there is an impressive amount of character required to attain an MD degree because of the massive commitment of time, the sacrifice of social life, and the delay of starting a family and making a living.

The average physician has no significant income until age thirty, and some much later than that. They live off the meager salaries that hospitals pay once they have started their postgraduate training, and most must moonlight and borrow money to make ends meet.

It's a sad commentary to me that entertainers and athletes, many of whom are drug addicts and criminals, certainly have not made similar commitments, and don't provide life-saving services, are held in such high esteem. It seems readily accepted that they make millions for rather mediocre performance, but a physician making one-tenth their income is considered rich and greedy.

There are many fine entertainers and athletes who give us much pleasure and do good works for the world, but they haven't put forth more effort toward developing their talents than the physician. One could also say that their art is much more pleasurable to practice than to spend hundreds of hours in a textbook, and the worst fate they can suffer isn't as bad as a patient dying under your care. A sour musical note or a dropped pass may be embarrassing or even cause your team to lose, but no one dies because of it.

I believe our priorities are in serious need of repair. I don't expect to be paid five million per year, but a physician's expertise is more valuable to humanity than a guy who sometimes catches a ball. I believe in the free enterprise system and don't advocate limiting the income of anyone, including athletes and entertainers, but don't allow business and government to denigrate the role of the physician to that of a skilled laborer unless you are prepared to accept the inconsistent results you receive.

I also believe airline pilots should be well paid, also dentists, veterinarians, nurses, paramedics, teachers, and a plethora of others who do a hell of a lot for this country and can't keep their job by batting 220, or raping a cheerleader.

The following stories are autobiographical sketches of real doctors who have been my partners in medicine and have some interesting histories of their own as well as some true personal experiences to relate.

Chapter 14
Cheating the Grim Reaper

At a well-seasoned age, it occurred to me that I have experienced a charmed life over the years. In the past, the grim reaper had several opportunities to snuff out my earthly existence.

At age two, I suffered from pneumonia. This disease killed more people than any other infectious disease in 1937, and there were no antibiotics or other effective treatments. The illness killed more children and elderly than healthy individuals. The doctor came to the house each day. In reality, there was little he could do other than give encouragement to my mother, but I survived without permanent ill effects.

At age 10, I had a bike accident that caused a serious head injury that rendered me, initially unconscious, and later left me confused and disoriented for two weeks. The same year, there occurred another head injury from an accidental baseball bat to my head while playing sandlot baseball.

At age 15, while fishing behind the dam at Balmorhea Lake in west Texas, I fainted for an unknown reason and floated downstream for a few minutes before a friend, Buddy Gray, dragged me out and threw me over a yucca plant. He beat on my back until, miraculously, I awoke, gagging and vomiting green algae-stained water. He saved my life. Drowning is, of course, deadly, but near drowning can also result in systemic abnormalities and severe pneumonia with lung damage. When the doctor later examined me, he admitted me to the hospital for two days and dismissed me without permanent damage.

A year later, while riding in a car driven by a teammate, Fuzz Herring, at 80 miles per hour on a two-lane highway between Kermit and Wink, Texas, an oncoming vehicle caused Fuzz to swerve, causing the car to hit the bar ditch. Again, we cheated the death angel as Fuzz negotiated the ditch and regained the highway without injury to anyone. I recall a cloud of dust that obscured the road behind us.

My senior year of football found me with multiple head injuries and concussions. I played in games that I never remembered and suffered headaches for years thereafter.

In 1959, while swimming in the Gulf of Mexico off a beach in Galveston, Texas, I had waded out in the surf until the water came to my neck. Deciding I had gone far enough, I started to swim back to the beach, but with each stroke I made no forward progress. Faster than I could swim toward shore a current, or riptide, carried me out to sea. I tried a few more times without success. Then I called, but my cries for help melted into the sound of noisy children playing on the beach. I paniced as the current took me farther out to sea. I couldn't touch bottom and had to tread water. Soon, I believed I would drown. Treading water until my legs became fatigued, I knew I would sink and die, if I didn't find the strength to swim to shore and live. Using all the willpower left in me, I swam with the urgency of a drowning man, and, miraculously, I made enough progress to touch bottom with my feet. This gave me a little time to rest, and by swimming and walking, I reached the shore, fatigued, but saved again.

As a practicing physician, I treated almost every infectious disease known to science: meningococcal meningitis, tuberculosis, encephalitis, Streptococcal and Staphylococcal diseases, and thousands of cases of influenza and other viral and bacterial illnesses. I only suffered the flu one time and strep throat once in all those years.

I have often wondered, did fate and happenstance keep me alive and functional or was there a Higher Authority that chose to keep me around for reasons known only to Him? Maybe He thought I might be a good doctor someday and help Him to save some lives?

Chapter 15
Barna Richards

As the third child, I was born to parents in the middle of the great depression. My father worked in a grocery store and my mother worked in a pecan distribution warehouse. They both felt fortunate to be employed in those difficult times. I stayed with my grandmother, along with my siblings. We were taught to respect authority, our parents, and other people. We were a church-going family, but not to the point of fanaticism.

My smart, talented, and industrious, older brother greatly influenced my life. He awoke every morning at four o'clock to deliver papers before school. He made good grades and was liked by everyone. In 1945, the day after graduation from high school, he went off to war. My pride for my big brother soared, but I was sick with fear that he might not come home alive. The day my brother left for duty, I couldn't tell him goodbye because I knew I would cry. Back in that time, boys did not cry. At my advanced age, I'm still saddened that I didn't tell my brother goodbye on that memorable day so many years ago. I loved him and was afraid he would be killed. Being a child at that time, I didn't have the emotional courage to tell him what he meant to me.

Thank God, the war ended shortly after my brother entered the military. He was coming home, alive, and without any wounds. I felt gloriously happy.

Our father never finished eighth grade, but he worked hard all his life. Ill or injured, he never missed a day on the job, except for the time the doctor insisted that he couldn't go to work with a ruptured appendix.

The only time I can remember him striking me consisted of a few tentative blows to the bottom when I was a child. I had stayed at the fishing hole way past curfew. My father was a quiet man who usually just agreed with mother. "What did your mother say?" was his usual response to a request from his children. A sensitive man, my father cried when he thought his children were in danger. He remained healthy until age ninety and never became senile, in spite of many years of smoking those little filterless cigarettes.

A bright high school graduate, my mother was much more than average for those times in rural Texas. She had a regal and proud persona and never would admit that her family was anything but first class, even though we were not among the economic elite. There were not many rich folks in the mid-thirties and forties. We were all in about the same boat...living frugally. People on welfare have many more luxuries today than the average person had fifty or sixty years ago. I remember being in awe of one of my friends who had a case of Coca-Cola at home. That family seemed extremely privileged. Most only had soft drinks at the drug store, and that constituted a rare treat. The average family didn't have the money for such frivolities. My friends and I sold coke bottles for two cents apiece or mowed lawns for a quarter to pay for our luxuries, such as movies or a trip to the ice cream parlor.

My mother owned a great zest for life and optimism that bordered on fantasy, always dreaming of something better for her family. She could have been a pioneer in a covered wagon but wished for a Cadillac. At age ninety, she still looked forward to each day as an opportunity to experience something new and exciting.

I inherited my mother's love of life, and, not wanting to miss any of it, I didn't sleep much. Mother thought I was near perfect. Because of that, I never wanted to bring disappointment or embarrassment to her or my family. Today, I give credit to my mother for believing in me. She is the reason for any success I have had. My mom and a few others who had confidence in me, more than I had in myself.

My older sister supported our parents emotionally and, sometimes, financially. She also inherited the strong work ethic typical of the children of the great depression and has been very successful in her endeavors as a businesswoman, wife, and mother.

Our younger brother had a kind and loving demeanor, always devoted to his family. He added great joy to our parents until he met with an early and tragic demise.

I took from my father the belief that work is essential to provide what one needs or wants in life. At the age of eight, I wanted to be a cowboy. In order to accomplish this, I had to dress like one and needed Levi's jeans which my mother detested.

"Only country hicks wear those things," she would say, and she refused to buy them. I took a paper route, saved my money, and bought my Levi's. As I slipped into the stiff denim material and admired the leather patch on the back, I thought myself a qualified rodeo man. This belief lasted a very short while. The bubble burst when I attempted to ride a bull. The experience terrified me as I spent more time flying into the air than I did on the bull's back. Needless to say, I didn't ride any more bulls and decided to be a drugstore cowboy instead.

In high school, academics played a secondary role to the other activities, but I did absorb more than my effort might indicate. I excelled in athletics, which captured the majority of my attention until I found the joys of the female gender. Sports and girls shared equal billing in my youth. I had the rare opportunity to play a significant role on a state championship football team. With this, the girls made me feel important and taught me how to kiss.

When I was fifteen years old, my parents moved from the little West Texas town of Wink. I didn't want to leave, to go to a new school. After all, I would lose a year of eligibility in sports. So I stayed and lived in a boarding house. I had no money and had to work as a janitor during the school year and in the oil fields in summer to pay room and board. The janitor work was not much fun, especially the girls' restrooms This disillusioned me since I had thought girls were sugar and spice and everything nice. However, the oil field work was exciting as well as character building. Bosses in that area of endeavor had no patience with laziness, but if a worker tried hard and kept busy, they treated us very well.

After graduation from high school, I entered college, not knowing exactly why but it seemed the thing to do. College didn't last long. I flunked out the first semester. The money I had made in the summer lasted until October, after that meals became a rarity. The grades were four Ds and one F. Someone said I spent too much time on one subject, but I wasn't certain which one it was.

That first college try wasn't time wasted. I met some students who seemed to know what they wanted in life. One was a pre-med student who worked night and day on his studies. Impressed with his labor, I began to understand that to accomplish anything, I would have to be much more committed. One of my high school classmates suffered a similar scholastic fate. He later became very successful and famous. He was Roy Orbison. We lived in the same rooming house in college, shared care packages from home, but mostly starved. When one parent sent a cake or other food, we all descended on it like a flock of vultures. One cake sat for a day or so and absorbed water like a sponge, there was no air conditioning, and the humidity was very high. That cake gave them several full stomachs, lying like a comforting bolus in the attenuated digestive tract. Roy went on to pursue his music career and has entertained the world with many top hits and beautiful songs. May he now rest in peace.

I felt as lost as a goose with blinders when I left college in the dead of winter. My means of transportation being the thumb. A classmate took me to Fort Worth. Then I had only three hundred and fifty miles farther to go. I stood in the rain and cold. Trucks splashed me with mud as they passed by and my lot in life seemed as low as one could get.

A hitchhiker is at the mercy of many fools and dangerous people. A young guy picked me up and drove as fast as the clunker could until I said, "This is as far as I'm going." It was a lie that probably saved my life. Another man stopped a few hours later and offered me a ride, which I reluctantly accepted, having no choice. The man was very kind and conversational. When he stopped at a café, he asked me what I wanted to eat.

"Oh, I'm not hungry," I replied.

"But son, I know you haven't eaten in several hours. You must be hungry."

"No, sir. Not a bit," I lied. The smell of food was painful, for I hadn't eaten in over two days. My pride wouldn't allow me to take a meal from a stranger. I didn't have a cent in my pocket. I hoped the kind man didn't notice the grumbling in my stomach. The remainder of the trip proved uneventful. I arrived home to parents who were very happy to see me, and me them. I had to move on because my parents couldn't solve my problems. I had to find my way in life and was having a bitch of a time doing it.

In the mid-fifties, with a recession raging and jobs almost non-existent, my big brother saved me by finding me a job. He also allowed me to live with his family. This was a life-saving event that I would never forget.

Those months with my brother and his wonderful family were happy times. Two small children who kept me entertained, playing canasta with the family, working hard, sleeping well, eating well, and having more time to think than any time since. This allowed me to make plans (only dreams at the time) for my life.

I decided to re-enter college and major in biology with pre-med aspirations, having no real confidence that I could accomplish what many considered to be one of the most demanding courses of study of that era.

The halcyon days with the family passed all too soon, and reality had to be recognized.

Returning to college in the fall of 1955, I found the pre-med curriculum to be very demanding and required all the self-discipline I could muster. However, determination, later obsession, with the quest to become a doctor pushed me toward my goal. Grades were the only important thing in my life. I studied until three or four o'clock every morning, and it didn't seem enough. Before long, the old nemeses of *poverty* and its buddy, *hunger*, returned to become my constant companions.

My walk home from class required passing by a hamburger stand, and the aroma of that glorious food caused great turmoil in my intestines. The fight between acid and the stomach lining became audible, and the acid won out. On some days when I felt I could barely walk to class from the ravages of hunger and self-pity, a strange thing happened. A sense of euphoria jumped into the brain as if I had taken a mind-altering drug, and the self-pity and fatigue temporarily left. It would be back, but this allowed respite from the misery for a while.

Joe Louis, one of my dearest friends, still laughs at the fact that I used to "steal" eggs from the landlady's chicken coop to ward off starvation. Her name was Mrs. McKinney, her rooming house appropriately called "McKinney House." She knew of the petty purloins and, knowing of my plight, occasionally offered me a meal. These occasions were tests of diplomacy because she ate like a petite bird and served bite-sized meals. My appetite of a nineteen-year-old man was equal to consuming the food, pots, pans, and utensils. However, I appreciated the thought. The most difficult part of these occasions was that she always wanted me to watch wrestling on TV after the meal. An avid fan, she became as vicious as an eighty pound, eighty-year-old woman could be when her favorite wrestler received one of those fake bashes in the head. She believed these were mortal wounds. She remains in my memory a kind woman, who was a factor in my journey on "doctor road." She took pride in her "boys."

I left after the spring semester, owing her four or five months rent, but I paid her back when I received my first paycheck from my summer job. She never complained, and always supported me. Mrs. McKinney became another miracle in my life.

Persistence paid off. I got a job as the keeper of the dispensary in the biology department. This put me in charge of all the equipment in the department and was a considerable responsibility. It also gave me credibility with the professors. I became a laboratory instructor, and this added to my meager income. It was infinitely better than the previous years of starvation. I could now eat. I bought a meal ticket each month and guarded it like the family jewels. Life was good. I had food and my grades became better—my confidence grew.

The glorious day came in the winter of 1959. I was accepted to medical school.

There isn't enough room at this time (or energy on my part) to tell the story of medical school in the '60s. While college students were protesting, smoking pot, defying their professors, and generally being unreliable, the medical student had no such luxuries. Some professors in medical school took pleasure in flunking a student out of school, and most students feared any attention that could be averse to his passing a course. Suffice it to say that fear of failure, and the ever-present poverty, resulted in diarrhea, vomiting, excessive alcohol (cheap) intake, and sleepless nights. The nights were really mornings because students never went to bed at night. My studies required being up way past midnight every night.

In 1961, the beginning of the third year, I did not have money for tuition. There were few loans then. My funds had been exhausted, and my hopes of continuing were fading when a friend told me of a wealthy benefactor who might be of assistance. I had little confidence of receiving help from a total stranger, but I had no alternative. In desperation, I picked up the phone and called Mr. Harris Kempner. Mr. Kempner possessed great wealth, a captain of industry who was well known but not perceived by many to be exceptionally charitable. Like many who have achieved greatness in business, many envied him and misunderstood him. With no credentials except desire and honesty, I was allowed to speak to Mr. Kempner. He listened to my story. I explained the fact that in my third year of medical school, I didn't have money for tuition, and would have to drop out if I didn't pay by the next week.

This gentleman asked that a letter be written, sent to him explaining the situation, and he would consider the request. I obtained stationary from a university secretary, wrote the letter, and mailed it within ten minutes of the conversation, expecting nothing. Within four days, I received a check for $500 with a note to sign, bearing no interest, to be paid when possible. I borrowed from Mr. Kempner several more times during my days as a student. After entering practice, as soon as I had the funds, the first debt I paid was Mr. Kempner. I'm forever grateful for the benevolence of this kind man who represents another of the miracles that occurred for me to become a physician.

Thousands of hours of study, many days of diarrhea and vomiting, constant fear of failure, frequent weekends of drunken stupor, and a lifestyle of no sleep or peace of mind, resulted in graduation with an M. D.

degree in 1963.

Two years later, as a young doctor, I finished my training to be a general practitioner, like Doc Adams of Gun Smoke fame. I entered practice with the same fear of failure with which I had entered pre-med and medical school, and I live with the same emotions to this day.

Because of the oppressive interference of government, attorneys, and HMOs, I gave up private practice in 1991, after twenty-six years of wonderful and meaningful relationships with thousands of great people. At this time, I was a full-time emergency physician who received my board certification in that specialty in 1988.

Chapter 16
Introduction to Frank Flory, MD

His friends call him "Uncle Frank," and he's one of the most unique individuals I've ever known. His young life wasn't easy, but I never saw him angry, never heard him yell at a nurse. He could walk on the hot coals of hell and not change his demeanor. He hates no one, not even the IRS, which took all of his retirement. Nor does he hold ill will toward his father who did him wrong as a child.

Dr. Flory was an orphan and lived in an orphanage as a child, yet he managed to succeed to achieve an MD degree. Today, he shows no evidence of rancor nor does he curse the system for being a victim of discrimination, although he was. He lives with the same principles that brought him to his station in life...hard work, day after day—sick, tired, or emotionally distraught. I know him to be a person who is reliable and, come hell or high water, he will come to your aid if you ask, or if you don't. At age sixty-three he continues to work nights, holidays, weekends, and in all states of mental turmoil and physical distress. He also was driven from private practice by the combined influences of government, HMOs, and litigious individuals, and is now a full-time emergency physician, working toward board certification. Learning never stopped in the medical profession.

When I think of people like Dr. Flory, and I hear sad

tales from those who just can't make it in life without government assistance, I become very frustrated and angry with our overprotective "leaders," who are so eager to pay for everything for everyone. Yes, Dr. Flory had many miracles in his life, as I did, but it was not luck. He put forth the work, set goals, and was very instrumental in making those miracles happen. He made a commitment early in life to be a doctor and worked and studied to do so. He easily could have blamed the system for his misfortunes and become a ward of the state, or a criminal, or worse, but he fought more hardships than the majority of welfare recipients today, and he has given back to society much more than his benefactors ever would have imagined. The same can be said for his brother, Don, who came from the depths of despair to become a provider of jobs and a solid citizen.

Take note, Mr. Jessie Jackson, it's work, education, and a strong resolve to succeed that make us rise above poverty and ignorance. It's true that there are those who need public assistance. I have experienced more hunger than most in society, and I don't wish that pain on anyone, but the reverse discrimination that you preach only causes more divisiveness and hatred. Your advice to young people encourages hostility, self-pity, and a belief that the world owes them something. The truth is that no one owes any of us anything. Father Beeman didn't owe Dr. Flory, and the people who aided me, neither did we expect anything, but we were willing to do the work expected of us to feel deserving of their benevolence. If I were in your position, Reverend Jackson, I would preach the old Mark Twainism "the harder I work, the luckier I get."

The following is Dr. Flory's story.

Chapter 17
Dr. Frank Flory's Story

I was born in a dumpy area of Kansas City, called Armordale, on May 24, 1933, to rather poor parents. My father was a cement finisher and an alcoholic. I later found out my mom was schizophrenic, yet extremely smart. In time, she wrote intelligent letters to me. As the oldest child, I had two brothers and two sisters and lived with my parents in Kansas City until I was nine years old —seven people in a four-room house that had only one water faucet. We bathed in a number two washtub, and our bathroom was an outhouse. The nicest thing I remember about the house was a swing on the front porch.

I used to get my brother to run off with me, and we had a habit of waiting in a field across from the house on Saturdays when our dad got paid. He always came home drunk, and while he was asleep, I would sneak in and take money from his pockets to get something to eat or go to the movies. One night after a raid on his wallet, my brother and I were in the movie when dad came in very angry and dragged us out. He took me to jail. I was nine years old.

I remember the cell was `steel-walled, with one window, and my cellmate was a guy more than twice my age and not very pleasant. After a time we started digging a hole in the roof of the cell, in an area secluded by the shower stall, trying to find a way out of the place.

We crawled into the ceiling but couldn't find an escape route. While we were scrambling around the attic the guard heard us, and we were caught. You may not believe this, but they put me in solitary confinement in a very small place about four by four feet, like in the movie "Papillion."

This turned out to be a blessing to me. My preacher, Mr, Hays found out what was happening, and wouldn't allow them to hold me any longer. He took me into his home and began to try to find someone to take me. By then I was considered a juvenile delinquent and wasn't a very desirable kid for adoption. He finally contacted the Juliet Fowler Home in Dallas and convinced them to take me. I remember being excited to be going to Texas with cowboys and Indians and buffalo and all the wild, wild west things that kids fantasize.

I was separated from my brothers and family, but things were much better for me in the home. We went to public schools and church outside the home. Even though I was considered a juvenile delinquent, I was a smart delinquent. This proved to be very beneficial to me because a doctor contacted the home and expressed his desire to help a deserving young person become a physician. As an eighth-grader, I thought this sounded pretty good. I took courses in science, math, and biology that would be helpful for me to go to medical school and graduated high school number 26 of 400.

Dr. Harrington, an eye, ear, nose, and throat physician, told me that if I made the grades in college to get into medical school, he would pay for my medical education. Of course, I had to go to college first, and that was not likely for a kid in an orphanage. Mr. Hays spoke to the congregation of the East Dallas Christian

Church, and two Sunday school classes agreed to send me all the way through college. One class gave me twenty-five dollars per month and the other thirty per month, which was a lot of money in those days, and they continued to send me this money until I graduated medical school. I graduated from Texas Christian University (TCU) cum laude and I'm still upset over one grade of "C" that I made in organic chemistry when I had a twenty-point average higher than some who were given the same grade that I received. That was the only "C" I made in college.

One of my closest friends in college was Charlie Bailey. Charlie took me home with him on weekends, and his father, who was a physician, often said to me,h "When you give nuthin'—you get nuthin' that's worth nuthin." I have reflected on those words many times and realize how true they are.

My counselor in pre-med told me I had the grades to go to medical school anywhere I desired. I chose Galveston because it was closer to home, the orphanage being the closest thing I had to a home. I still felt a lot of affection for Mr. Hays and some of the matrons there and wanted to be close enough to visit on occasion. I'm forever grateful for the care and support they gave me over the years.

Medical school separates the real achievers from the impostors, and I managed to cram four years into five, having to repeat the third year because of overconfidence and too many extracurricular activities. I became serious again and graduated without any further problems. It's a very sobering experience to repeat a year of medical school.

One of my classmates had a 1947 Chrysler, and

since he lived in Dallas I hitched a ride home with him on holidays. Now, it's three hundred miles from Galveston to Dallas, and our all-time record for this trip was under four hours. I was probably lucky to survive some of those rides.

I did my internship at St. Joseph's Hospital in Fort Worth, and one of the things I will always regret is that I didn't do a specialty residency, but I chose to go into practice after my internship because I needed to make money and pay back all I owed and make a living for myself. I tried private practice for a while with some doctors in east Texas who wanted to use me as their night, weekend, and holiday slave for minimum wage and soon became disenchanted with that arrangement.

I then went into practice with two doctors in Euless, Texas, both of whom are friends to this day, but I eventually opened my own office where I practiced until 1978 when I moved my practice to Arlington, Texas. I remained in private practice there until 1993 when I was asked to become a full-time emergency physician at the hospital where I'm now employed.

I have been involved with the emergency room at Arlington Memorial Hospital since 1970 when a group of family doctors and surgeons formed Physicians Emergency Group, an organization that provided physicians for emergency room coverage for twenty years. I remember that I had the inaugural shift after the formation of this group. We worked the office during the day and the ER once or twice per week at night. The nights we worked the ER required us to be up without sleep for about thirty-six hours. In addition, some of us delivered babies, and some were surgeons who were also up many nights doing emergency surgery. Sleep was a rare commodity for us. Insane?

The stories of my siblings are interesting for several reasons. My brother, Don, was put into an orphanage at age eleven. Father Don Beeman came to his rescue, also, because brother Don had gotten into some difficulties, and Father Beeman found a place for him in a boys home in Kansas. He graduated high school, went to college at TCU, and later got his Masters and PhD degrees in chemistry. He now has his own business and is much more financially secure than his physician older brother.

I had not seen my brother in many years when we finally got together. One of my most memorable occasions occurred when Don invited me and my wife, Kate, to spend a weekend with him and his wife, Norma, at their cabin outside of Austin. The Austin hill country of Texas is one of the most beautiful places in the world. We ate steaks and drank a fifth of Wild Turkey. The amazing thing was that neither of us got drunk. We reminisced most of the night over our previous escapades as kids and were both grateful, and somewhat puzzled, that two kids with such shaky beginnings could be in the relatively lofty positions we now occupied.

My other siblings did not fare as well as Don and myself. It's of some interest that of the five children, two are doctors—one a physician, the other a PhD in chemistry. The others were of a different mix. Little sister, Lana Sue, has the intelligence of a third grader and requires custodial care, while my other sister can care for herself. The younger brother is of average intelligence. All of this can probably be explained by the knowledge I learned much later in life that my father and mother were second cousins.

All said and done, I guess I'm lucky to have come to

this point in life. A little kid who grew up in a home with one water faucet and an outside toilet, a nine-year-old jailbird, and attempted-escapee with the chance of a snowball in hell of ever making anything of himself became a doctor.

One of my more interesting experiences in the emergency room involved a patient who came to the ER after being assaulted with a knife. She was alert and oriented, laughing and talking with her friends, and very drunk. I examined her and told her that she needed some X-rays and some sutures in her forehead where she had a horizontal laceration that was similar to a surgical incision. She protested that she couldn't afford to pay for private care and preferred to go to the county hospital. At that time, it was politically correct to do this, and she was allowed to go to John Peter Smith Hospital in Fort Worth. I received a call the next day from JPS, and the resident who cared for her told me that, not only did she have a laceration of her forehead, but she also had a knife blade in the frontal lobe of her brain. A neurosurgeon removed the blade, and she did just fine. I guess her frontal lobe was so soaked with alcohol that she didn't know the difference.

Another incident, somewhat humorous, occurred when a nurse came to me and said that a male patient had something stuck in his rectum. The nurses always had a tendency to bring these types of problems to the male physicians if we were working with a female doctor. It so happened that I was working with Dr. Jane Torgerson, and when she overheard the nurses dialogue, she said, "Oh! Let me do it. I have smaller hands." Well, Dr. Torgerson came back with her face flushed with success. She had removed a vibrator from the rectum of this hapless individual, and both were relieved that the ordeal was over. “Torgy” is another story. She seemed to get more of these hidden treasures than the rest of us.

Chapter 18
Introduction to Hoyt Frenzel, MD

Dr. Frenzel succeeded me as medical director of the ER at Arlington Memorial Hospital in 2007. I can't think of anything that could have pleased me as much as it did for him to be the new director. He accomplished more in a few weeks than I could have done in years—establishing AMH as a certified heart center, and, later, as a stroke center. This required the blessing of the hospital, and then cardiologists had to be willing, or coerced, to be on call for cardiac catheterization on short notice. The cath lab had to be readily available, and all had to be done in a definite and established time-frame.

The stroke center requirements were similar and required neurologists to be available. This may not seem such a great achievement to the casual observer, but my long years of trying to effect change in doctor's habits caused me frustration, headaches, and heartburn. This all points to the fact that Dr. Frenzel is a very effective leader.

Dr. Frenzel not only brought about needed change to the system, but his patient care exceeded expectations, as he provided impeccable care to them as well. During my term as director, I can't recall a single complaint toward him from patients, medical or nursing staff, or administration. This is unique because there is always someone who will complain even when everything is done perfectly.

After reading his bio, one can see that Dr. Frenzel, MD, FACEP, FAAEM, is an extraordinary person, an excellent physician, a talented innovator, and a very effective leader of men. My personal experience as medical director taught me that "leading" doctors can be similar to herding cats. They were all "smarter" than me-which might be true, but sometimes there are too many chiefs and not enough Indians. Dr. Frenzel accomplished this task with much less conflict from the ER doctors than I did. His leadership ability exceeded mine. That isn't humble pie on my part--it's a fact.

The same corporation that relieved me of the position of medical director also replaced Dr. Frenzel. The difference is that he did more in ten years that I accomplished in twenty. Furthermore, I was 72 years old, tired, burnt out, and had few innovative ideas. Forty-two years in the same ER, and twenty years as medical director might burn anyone out. On the other hand, Dr. Frenzel still possessed abundant energy, talent, and desire to continue the successes he had initiated.

The corporation bases their decisions on numbers. Patient satisfaction scores are the benchmark of their decision-making process. These scores can, and are, "gamed" by some of the hospitals in the system by deleting certain areas that show poor scores and keeping the positive responses. Dr. Frenzel had the business acumen to fudge the numbers, but his honesty and Christian beliefs didn't allow that.

I'm sure that the new ER group is comprised of excellent physicians, but I doubt they will ever find a medical director to equal Dr. Frenzel's talent and leadership skills.

I appreciate Dr. Frenzel's kind words towards me. The following is his story.

Chapter 19
Dr. Hoyt Frenzel's Story

I was born in Minnesota, and then we moved to Texas in 1976. An average middle-class family, my father was a journalist who worked in the merchandise and travel incentive industry, and my mother was a homemaker and raised the kids.

My parents valued and stressed the importance of getting high-quality education. We moved to the suburbs of Arlington, Texas with great new schools and with teachers like my English teacher, Mrs. Alice Peterson, who were passionate about teaching. In the beginning, my parents incentivized (bribed) the kids with report card money and for reading books. $10 for each "A," $5 for each "B", nothing for C's. If we made a "D" or God forbid an "F," we'd owe them big. Little did I know, or understand at the time, that these learning incentives subconsciously fueled my passion and hunger for learning, Later my perseverance led me to become a physician. My brother also became triple-boarded in Surgery, Bariatric, and Cosmetic Surgery. At that time, no other members of our family were doctors or worked in the medical profession. Fast forward, 25 years later, Mrs. Peterson was our lead volunteer at the hospital that I worked for and assisted me with an ER expansion project.

I was introduced early in life to medicine through the direct observation of my grandmother's health struggles.

My grandmother, Wilma Frenzel, was diagnosed at a young age with Parkinson's Disease. It robbed her of her health during the prime of her life. Because of her rapidly advancing disease, she volunteered for a medical study at Mayo Clinic in Rochester, Minnesota. She was one of the first patients to undergo an experimental brain surgery in an attempt to transplant dopamine cells back into the Substantia Nigra, the area of the brain destroyed by the disease. Unfortunately, the procedure was not successful. As the years went by, the disease progressed. She later died of complications from her disease while visiting us in Texas.

I later learned that Parkinson's Disease robs the nervous system of the body's ability to coordinate fine motor movements. The classic Tim Conway "shuffling gait" and "masked facies" or loss of facial expressions are the hallmarks of the disease. While visiting us in Texas, she tripped walking, fell, and hit her head. She died at Arlington Memorial Hospital, a hospital that would be important to me later in my life, the very hospital, in the same ER, where I took my first job after residency, and where I later succeeded Dr. Barna Richards as the Medical Director. Reflecting back, witnessing her personal and daily struggles fueled my intense desire to learn everything I could about the human body and later about medicine. My parents started their own company. It grew over the years. I worked on and off at the company on a part-time basis. I learned everything from shipping and receiving to accounting. My father had a team of salesmen. He was (and still is) one of the most amazing leaders, motivators, and mentors that I've ever met. One of his salesmen was an ex-Dallas Cowboy who played in the Super Bowl. Meeting and working with him gave me a great insight into success. Real success on a global scale. I recall one of his pearls of wisdom: “At the end of the day, all you have is your reputation. Your word is gold.” Words I would later live my career by.

Over the years, I basically got a real-world MBA and was able to grow with the family company. I attended the University of North Texas (UNT) and took some business classes but found them dry and not realistic like the experience that I obtained working. Over the years, the company grew to 20+ employees and was doing millions of dollars a year in sales. I studied biology and chemistry and became very interested in considering medicine as a career. I graduated cum laude with a straight 4.0 in all my biology classes.

After seeing many mediocre pre-med students that “brown-nosed” the deans to get into medical school, I became disenfranchised with the bureaucratic process of going directly into medical school. I decided I wanted to take a year off. I worked full-time for our family business. One year turned into three-and-a-half. I started a new division of the company. We created safety incentive programs to keep employees safe and to prevent on-the-job injuries. We sold them to companies like TGI Fridays, American Airlines, Xerox, and Sky Chefs. We did one million dollars in sales our first year. I employed and managed a few friends and some employees that worked for me. It was a great life and leadership opportunity. Before I knew it, I was running my own business inside the family business. I was able to work on large projects for many of the Fortune 500 companies in the DFW metroplex. I was blessed to work with some of the most amazing leaders in business in the area.

On my time off, I took EMT (Emergency Medical

Technician) classes. At night, I rode out on the ambulance and earned my EMT certification. This exposed me to real-world medicine.

While in Bermuda on a business trip with my father, I was reflecting on my life. I was immensely grateful for the opportunities given to me and for the life experiences. But inside, after deep reflection and introspection, I realized I needed to be truly fulfilled. I had to be honest and truthful with myself. I knew, deep inside, my calling was medicine. Yes, I was being groomed to take over the family business, but I knew I needed to pursue my calling. After deep contemplation and discussion with my father, he told me to apply to medical school and follow my dreams.

I re-read all my chemistry, biology, physics, and biochemistry books. I worked all day and took the Princeton Review (online tutoring) at night to prepare. I took graduate level biochemistry and pharmacology classes at UNT, taught by the very same teachers that taught the same subjects at the UNT Medical School in Fort Worth. I aced the classes. I literally broke the class curve. Other students voiced their disdain. That only fueled my passion to work harder and prepare for medical school. I took the MCAT (Medical College Admission Test), did med school interviews and got in the next year.

My life was on autopilot. Fueled by a passion to learn. armed with real-world life experience, combined with a strong business background, my journey began. I went to medical school at the University of Texas Health Science Center San Antonio (UTHSC). I was president of my class. I immediately put to use my entrepreneurial and business skills. I wrote a study manual on neuroanatomy and histology. We bound them up and sold them for a class fundraiser. We made class videos and started a scribe service. We created logoed t-shirts, hats, and sweatshirts and sold them for four years. My business experience paid off big. While at UTHSC, I met my wife and soulmate.

I attended East Carolina's Pitt County Memorial Hospital for Emergency Medicine Training. I picked that program because it was one of the very first EM residency programs. The ER doctors ran the entire hospital. The Dean of the Medical School chaired the department, and ER docs chaired every major department. It was perfect—another real-world MBA in administration while learning Emergency Medicine. During residency, I was the Chief Resident and served as the student delegate for the State of North Carolina to the American Medical Association. We went to Washington and I learned about lobbying.

My first job after residency was at Texas Health Arlington Memorial Hospital in the Emergency Department. While there, Dr. Richards took me under his wing and mentored me. I was slowly introduced to hospital committee work, process improvement and the business side of medicine. After Dr. Richards retired, I was asked to assume the role of Medical Director and was blessed with ten years of service to my community in that role.

I always saw medicine as my calling. In my new job, I wanted to give back to the community that raised and educated me, using my background and business acumen to do it. I persevered for the next ten years working as hard as I could to accomplish that goal.

One day while working in the emergency department, my old high school English teacher checked in for treatment. Mrs. Peterson had retired from teaching and soon became lead volunteer at our hospital. She was the interior decorator at the hospital. She was in charge of all holiday and special event decorations. That day the small ER was overcrowded. There were no beds. I felt very guilty and personally responsible. When she got to a room, I apologized for the delay. We dreamed of a larger facility. One that would better serve the community that we lived in. We later pitched the idea to the CEO and Board of Directors. They approved an ER expansion. We raised multiple millions from the community. Mr. Robinson of the Amon Carter Foundation put a one million dollar check in my hand for the project. Wow! We were off to the races. We nearly doubled the size of the ER, including twenty new treatment rooms, an eight-bed fast track, a new waiting room, and trauma/critical care beds.

After expansion came a rush of quality improvement projects. First was capital and equipment to modernize our facility. Then later came accreditation projects - merit badges of quality. The first project was creating a Primary Stroke Center and next, a Chest Pain Center with PCI (Percutaneous Intervention, Angioplasty, with heart catheterization lab and equipment). The following year was Acute Heart Failure. Then, Atrial Fibrillation with EP (electrophysiology), very specialized equipment and specially trained cardiologists to map electrical heart conduction abnormalities and treat them with surgical interventions. At that time, we had one of only a few Hansen machines in the country for cardiac mapping. This later spawned the Texas Health Heart and Vascular Hospital, a joint venture between THR (Texas Health Resources), the cardiologists, and vascular surgeons. Despite their hard work and accreditation, ER physicians were not allowed to invest in the project.

Next was "Own the Bone," an orthopedic accreditation. Later "Cancer Accreditation" by the Joint Commission. In 2016, came Trauma Level 3 Accreditation by the American Academy of Surgeons. Along the way, I was able to be the lead physician for the Cotton Bowl games and fans attending games at the Cowboy stadium and the Nation Championship playoffs. When Arlington hosted Super Bowl XVL, since my hospital and ER was literally a few blocks down the street from the stadium, we were involved with FBI and Homeland Security tabletop drills. When dignitaries came into town, we developed plans with the Secret Service and law enforcement for dignitary protection and care plans.

June 1, 2017, came hard. I was fired. Politely asked to step down for a new group to take over. Our democratic group of twenty-five physicians was dismissed after over thirty years of service in time for a mega-group to take over. Apparently, our ED throughput metrics and patient satisfaction data were not where it needed to be. Despite many warnings and efforts to improve the metrics, we just did not move the needle enough for the administrators. It's big corporate business—to the tune of four billion dollars a year. I soon learned from big business that there is no loyalty for service. No respect for altruistic motives. Little care for hard work, or giving back to others. To the MBA and company men, it's all about metrics and data. No matter how absurd. Regardless of impact on outcomes or patient care. Unfortunately, the bureaucracy of medicine, although riddled with good intentions, is now about using pre-written order-sets and protocols. About following the rules to meet the metrics. About bypassing physician judgment and experience. So, I ask you: Is this wise? Is this the measure of quality? Are we doing no harm?

Regardless, after sixteen years of service, I'm reminded that I've saved many lives—many that I will remember forever. Some lives, despite our very best care, we couldn't save. Some that continue to haunt me.

Over that period, our ER saw an average of 70,000 patients a year. I estimate that over that time, I was directly or indirectly involved in the care of over 1.2 million patients—including friends and family, a whopping twenty-plus million. That's a truly blessed career. That's my life's work and I would not change a second for I know that God directs my every step.

Finally, I would like to thank all those that mentored and molded me into what I am.

To prior our leaders and pioneers in the field of Emergency Medicine, like Dr. Barna Richards.

To the appendices (interns and residents) of our trade. May you continue to grow the profession.

Chapter 20
Introduction to Roy Yamada, MD

In our ER, Dr. Yamada was what might be called a clean-up man, like the fourth batter in baseball, who is usually the best hitter and expected to bring home the teammates on base. As our clean-up man, he very efficiently and effectively treated more patients than any of the rest of us, thus, cleaning the bases—the backlog of waiting patients.

Dr. Yamada told me he developed a liking for the southern mainland lifestyle, so much so, that upon graduating medical school, he sought training in orthopedic surgery at John Peter Smith Hospital in Fort Worth, Texas.

Dr. Yamada felt great compassion for his patients. Many incidents exemplify even more compassion for those of lesser means. In the years before government programs became commonplace, most doctors gave much of their time to charity care without fanfare or the general public's knowledge. Dr. Yamada often gave to those in need of medicines.

He served our ER in excellent fashion for a number of years. Due to his passion for pre-hospital care and working with paramedics, he served as medical director for various EMS organizations and is a superior mentor for young paramedics.

Chapter 21
Dr. Roy Yamada's Story

I was raised on a seven-acre farm, growing corn, tomatoes, green beans, watermelon, etc. I guess you'd call it a garden by Texas standards. Growing up in Hawaii meant hearing the stories of December 7th, 1942. My grandmother often told the story of seeing the planes flying over the Island to drop the bombs that began the United States' involvement in World War II

At age seven I wanted to be a doctor. Our country doctor, Dr. Yanagi, had polio at a very young age, sentencing him to life in a wheelchair. He was a great person, and I wanted to do what he did. So, I attended the University of Hawaii and had great professors from all over the USA. After graduating, I decided on Orthopedic Surgery and spent a year in General Surgery at the University of Hawaii. I graduated in 1980.

As a boy, I owned a silver transistor radio and I listened to my favorite station. It played country music, the only station that played country. It was the closest music I could find to Hawaiian music with the steel guitar and slow singing. When it came time to pick a residency, orthopedics in my case, I wanted west or south, California and Texas, nothing east or north. That's why I did my external at John Peter Smith Hospital. I chose JPSH and loved the Texas people and the culture—slower than Hawaii. And I could listen to country music 24/7. After my senior internships in orthopedics in California and then in Texas at John Peter Smith Hospital (JPSH) in Fort Worth, I developed a liking for the Texas indigent. In Hawaii, there's only private hospitals and no county or public hospitals operating on a single-payer system that was overseen by the state of Hawaii.

On "Match Day," I marched with JPSH Orthopedic Surgery and went through a rotating internship. While on the surgery rotation, one of my patients had a ruptured ovarian cyst that had been explored and washed out and left open to heal by secondary retention. I changed her dressing twice a day, One day, on my first round, I noticed a black mass on her lower lip. I inquired about it, and she said, "It's dip!" I had never seen it before.

Another incident that occurred years ago at JPS ER was the time I treated a child with congestion, cough, fever, ear infection, and general malaise. I gave the young, first-time mom, instructions about fever, fluids and directions to see a doctor the next day, then I gave her prescriptions for antibiotic and cough medication. She told me that she had no money to buy the medications. I then called a pharmacy and asked the pharmacist to fill the prescriptions and charge it to my account. The pharmacist said he couldn't do that because, if he did this for one patient he had to do it for everyone. This apparently related to some federal mandate of which none of us doctors were aware. Knowing the child really needed the medication, I gave the mom money for the prescriptions.

JPS fit me. I liked the fact due to its mission as a "charity" hospital. Before finishing the ortho residency, I decided that emergency medicine was my destiny.

Then, after concentrated study, I passed the arduous tests to become board certified in the specialty.

Chapter 22
Introduction to Bohn Allen, MD

Dr. Bohn Allen joined a group of twenty physicians in 1970 who agreed to provide doctors to treat patients in the ER at Arlington Memorial Hospital. He provided this service for a number of years until he found that working all night in the ER and performing surgery at 7:00 a.m. was not a healthy combination.

To enumerate all of Dr. Allen's achievements and awards would require a book larger than this one. He set an example for all physicians to emulate, and he did all this with cheerful confidence that gained him respect and close relationships with his fellow physicians.

Chapter 23
Dr. Bohn Dixon Allen's Story

I was born on October 15, 1935, in Alpine, Texas, a small west Texas town in the Big Bend region not far from the Rio Grande River in the middle of the "Great Depression" when life was difficult at best. I was the first-born of two sons to William C. Allen, Jr. and Margaret G. Scudday. As teenagers too young to get married in Texas, my parents eloped from Alpine to Carlsbad, New Mexico, in December of 1933 where they were married by a Justice of the Peace.

After my birth, my father went to the County Clerk's office to fill out the birth certificate because they couldn't agree on what to name me at birth. My father wanted to name me Bohn after an all-American halfback at the University of Texas in 1935. Against the wishes of my mother and both grandmothers, my dad filled out the paper and named me "Bohn." By the time everyone learned about it, it was too late to change it. My paternal grandmother, not one to be trifled with, declared I would be called "Dickie" and the name stuck until I left for college. Once I left Alpine, I was known as Dick or Bohn depending on how well one knew me. Most of the professors referred to me as "Bone" instead of Bohn.

Except for two years, from 1943 to 1945, when my father joined the Army Air Corps to train as a WWII bomber pilot, I lived in Alpine. Having to move frequently, my parents decided to leave me with my maternal grandparents in Fort Stockton, Texas.

Early in 1946, after the end of WWII, my father separated from the service and returned to Alpine to go into business for himself. I returned to Alpine and lived with my parents and brother until 1953 when my father sold his business and moved to Midland, Texas, to become a commercial pilot for an oil company. My father never got flying out of his system.

Being involved in sports and pursuing a basketball scholarship to Texas Tech University in Lubbock, Texas, I wanted to stay in Alpine to finish my senior year in high school to play in the basketball and football seasons. I finished high school living with friends who had two sons involved in sports and earned room and board working in their grocery store and doing chores around the house.

In my early years, I grew up around my father's dry cleaning business which was located next door to a hospital belonging to a general surgeon who also did family practice. Waiting for my parents to close the shop each evening, I spent many hours playing doctor in back of the hospital. I knew early that I wanted to be a doctor, and more specifically a surgeon.

Instead of pursuing the scholarship to Texas Tech, I decided to go to the University of Texas (UT) in Austin to get a pre-medical education, hoping to improve my chances of getting into medical school. I applied and was accepted to UT in August of 1954.

After enrolling in UT, I was still interested in playing basketball. So I tried out for the freshman team and made it. I enjoyed playing for UT and was offered a half-scholarship (tuition and books) for my sophomore year. However, after the team made an extended road trip early in the season, I missed several classes and labs in organic chemistry, embryology, and comparative anatomy. I realized I would never catch up if I missed any more classes, especially labs. I had to forego basketball and focus on my studies to get into medical school in three years instead of four. I had limited resources and worked two to three jobs to pay my way.

I reached my goal, completing all of my premedical requirements in three years, and passed the Medical College Aptitude Test (MCAT) examination. I applied to the University of Texas-Medical Branch in Galveston, Texas, and was accepted, enrolling in September of 1957.

After completing my freshman year of medical school, I met and married Ann Cecile Thoman, a nursing student in the degree nursing program. After a short courtship, we were married in December of 1958 during the holiday break and have remained married and devoted to each other for the past fifty-nine years.

Throughout medical school and nursing school Ann and I each had two or three jobs. We were the only means of support to get each other through medical and nursing school and never considered student loans fearing we wouldn't be able to pay them back. Amazingly, we finished school able to leave Galveston free of any student debt. In fact, when we left Texas to start my internship in Denver, Colorado, we were free of debt, had money in the bank, had a new car, and a new baby girl.

In 1959, I joined the U.S. Army student program and was commissioned a Second Lieutenant on active duty. This allowed us to receive a second lieutenant's pay, housing allowance, commissary and PX privileges, and helped our finances considerably. Ann had finished nursing school and worked as a nurse in Labor and Delivery at John Sealy Hospital in Galveston. Upon graduation from UTMB, we were assigned to Fitzsimons Army Hospital in Aurora, Colorado to begin my internship.

After completing my internship, I decided to continue my military career and accepted a general surgery residency at Madigan Army Hospital in Tacoma, Washington. We spent four years there.

When I completed my surgery residency in 1966, a representative from the Surgeon General's Office in Washington, DC came to visit the graduating residents to inquire what their interest and preference for their next assignment might be. When the colonel asked me where I would like to go, I told him I wanted to go to Fort Hood in Killeen, Texas. The colonel got a stunned look on his face and exclaimed that in all of his years in the Surgeon General's Office he had never had anyone request Fort Hood. I assured him that there would be no problem being assigned to Fort Hood.

After serving one year at Fort Hood, I was reassigned to the Surgical Research Unit (SRU) at Brooke Army Medical Center (BAMC) in San Antonio, Texas, to do a fellowship in a new treatment of burn patients. The SRU was the Burn Center for all severe burn patients of all military services. The Army planned to send me to Japan to establish an offshore burn unit to treat Vietnam burn casualties. It would be the burn center for the Far East Command.

I arrived in Japan at the 106th General Hospital in Yokohama, Japan, in June of 1967. The hospital was converted from a group of buildings used to train police trainees into a 1000-bed general hospital. It actually was well suited for the hospital conversion. The large open wards were conducive to caring for large numbers of patients. Assigned as Chief of General Surgery and the Director of the Burn Unit, I was responsible for the establishment of the Burn Center using a new burn treatment with sulfamylon, a sulfa-based cream, to control burn wound infection. As chief of the surgery service, I cared for thousands of war casualties in addition to the burn patients.

One of the main duties I had was to work with the Air Force of the Far East Command to establish a safe air-evacuation system to evacuate acutely burned patients from Vietnam to Japan. Once the severely burned patients were completely stabilized, they were then evacuated to the SRU at BAMC. Most other burn-patients were treated and skin grafted and transferred back home to a military hospital close to their home.

After three years, and treating over three thousand burn-patients and multiple other war casualties, I was reassigned to Letterman Army Hospital in San Francisco, California as Chief of General Surgery in charge of training surgery residents and medical students.

I completed my payback time of five years to the Army in 1971, to settle my obligation for medical school and residency training. I decided to resign my commission and separate from the Army to begin a private practice of surgery. Ann and I started looking for a place to settle down and build a practice. We initially considered returning to the Seattle area where we had been for my surgical residency, but we wanted to look at possible opportunities in Texas. We were both homesick after being gone for ten years.

We made trips to West Texas, the panhandle of Texas and the Midland-Big Spring area. Then we wanted to visit the Fort Worth, Dallas, and Arlington area to take the kids to Six Flags Over Texas. I contacted a good friend from childhood who was an attorney in Arlington. He introduced me to three surgeons, the mayor, and a hospital administrator. It was quite an introduction to Arlington. Ann and I thought it was definitely an opportunity.

When we returned to San Francisco, we had already received several packets of information from the mayor covering real estate home listings, schools, and information from the city planning department. One of the surgeons we met called and expressed his need for a partner or associate. After a second visit to Arlington, we determined it would be a good place to start a surgical practice. In March of 1971, after separating from the Army, we moved to Arlington to begin a new life.

Beginning a new practice is difficult at first. I volunteered to cover the emergency room. It was a good way to meet the local physicians and to develop a referral base for patients. I camped out in the ER to accept any patients I was asked to treat. It proved to be a good way to build a practice.

At about the same time, a group of family physicians and surgeons decided to form a group to cover the emergency room at Arlington Memorial Hospital. This group agreed to see the patients who came to the ER and either treat them or screen them and call their personal physician for instructions. It was actually a pretty good system at that time for patients, the doctors, and the community. It eliminated a lot of waiting and delays in treatment. The patients, for the most part, liked it. It gave the ER some degree of continuity in care.

As time passed, the doctors formed a limited professional corporation, known as Physician's Emergency Group (PEG) to do the administrative, billing, and legal functions for the group. Most of the income generated was supposed to go to an investment plan for the retirement of the doctors. Over the first two to three years it seemed to work out to some degree because no one was taking any reimbursement from the group or the invested funds. The group did decide to invest in a condominium in Crested Butte, Colorado, to be used by the members of PEG or rented if no one was using it. That seemed like a good idea at the time but later became unworkable.

After a few years, the accounting of the corporation became problematic and the members were not sure where all the money and investments were located. It was unclear where the retirement funds were held. Eventually, the group disbanded and most of the doctors never realized much for their time spent working in the ER. The good news for me was that I became known in the community and became established in Arlington. Working with the family doctors and meeting other physicians in the community helped me develop a good referral base which was invaluable over the years I was in practice. What I learned from the experience was that I couldn't work all night in the ER and still see patients and operate the next day. I decided it was best to take care of my own patients and leave the ER coverage to other physicians.

Over the years, I went on to participate in organized medicine and my specialty societies. I was a founding member and President of the Arlington Medical Society

(AMS), President of the Tarrant County Medical Society (TCMS), President of the Fort Worth Surgical Society (FWSS), President of the Texas Medical Association (TMA), and President of the Texas Surgical Society (TSS).

I was honored to receive the Gold-Headed Cane from TCMS, the Ashbel Smith Distinguished Alumni Award from UTMB and the Distinguished Service Award from TMA. I was a founding member of the Board of Trustees of Texas Health Resources Health Care System and Chair of the Board of Trustees of Arlington Memorial Hospital. I always considered my greatest honor was to serve God, my patients, medicine, the hospital, and my community.

Anecdotal Stories from the ER

I always volunteered to take call on New Year's Eve so I could spend Christmas with my family. One New Year's Eve a patient came to the ER with a severe laceration to his wrist. This man had a history of overdoing the celebration of the New Year and drinking a little too much. On one particular night, the patient decided to stay home and put up a tent in the backyard to camp out with his kids to celebrate the New Year. Unfortunately, he was carving a stake to anchor his tent and the knife slipped, cutting his wrist and severing multiple tendons, a nerve, and an artery. After a prolonged operation to repair all of the damage, he awakened in the recovery room and looked around and exclaimed, "Damn it, I knew I should have partied it up last night!"

There was another memorable patient who came to the ER periodically after fighting. He was a classic "redneck" who would just as soon fight as drink beer, although he did both regularly. Over the years, I had sutured him up many times and had become his personal surgeon. On this occasion, he arrived in the ER with a broken nose and several lacerations of his face and hand. After repairing all of the damage, I asked him what had happened. The patient broke out in a big grin and said, "Doc, you think I'm bad, you ought to see that other SOB!" We both laughed and the patient left the ER to fight another day.

Chapter 24 Introduction to Joseph Delprincipe, D.O.

Dr. Delprincipe joined our group, AEMA, and very soon became a valuable asset. He assumed leadership positions in the ER, becoming president of the group, and he became Chief of Staff of the hospital. This was unusual in that ER doctors aren't commonly elevated to the level of chief of staff. He describes in his bio some of the difficulties ER doctors face when dealing with administrators. This is more problematic with the takeover of medicine by large corporations that are directed by accountants rather than those providing the care. I expect this trend will continue.

Chapter 25
Dr. Joseph Delprincipe's Story

I grew up in upstate NY in the '70s in a farming community. Back in those days, I was an avid runner in high school and college, running many 10K, 20K, and several marathons. Life was simple. I competed on the rifle team and shot at various competitions. We even carried our twenty-two rifles in a case on the school bus, something you could never do today.

After graduation from high school, I went to the State University of New York (SUNY) at Fredonia in New York, a music school. I was a bassoonist and studied under Ron Daniels from the Buffalo Philharmonic. After three years in college in music, Christmas of 1977, during the New York blizzard, I decided I needed to change my major to chemistry. So with my soon-to-be wife and one child on the way, I graduated with a BS in chemistry, then left for a PhD program in chemistry at the University of North Texas (UNT) in Denton, Texas.

I got into medical school at the Texas College of Osteopathic Medicine (TCOM) in Fort Worth, which I attended from 1979 - 1983. I graduated in 1983 from TCOM and did a rotating internship, then entered the practice track for Emergency Medicine and became board certified by the American Board of Emergency Medicine (ABOEM). There weren't that many residency programs back then, especially for DOs. I worked for several companies in EM in the North Texas area.

(Coastal, Spectrum, Shoemauker, etc.)

In early ER days, emergency room companies came and went, but the ER doctors stayed on many times. I worked at Campbell Memorial in Weatherford, Texas, and Palo Pinto General Hospital in Mineral Wells, Texas, then landed an ER job at Dallas/Fort Worth Medical Center. In the early 80s, that place was a thriving hospital with many residency programs (OB/GYN, Surgery, Family Practice, Internal Medicine). It was a mixed-staff hospital of MDs and DOs. I eventually left and joined Dr. Pratho and Dr. Weaver, who owned Texas Emergency Medicine Physicians (TEMP), an ER group in Arlington.

I also worked at Medical Center in Arlington (MCA). I worked my way up the chain and became the medical director. Then everything changed, and Questcare took over all the Hospital Corporation of American (HCA) hospitals. That was my first experience with a corporate takeover of ER groups. I was told nothing would change. OMG! That was BS! I knew for many years ER contract groups were making lots of money off the back of ER doctors.

The most wonderful thing happened to me one day at MCA. That was when the entire emergency staff spoke up to Questcare and said, "Under no circumstances did they want me to leave.

Eventually, I did leave when the Arlington Emergency Medical Associates (AEMA) at Arlington Memorial Hospital (AMH) recruited me. That was the best thing that ever happened to me. Over the years, I became the president of AEMA and continued to be the president until another ER group took over AEMA. We transformed into a well-known group of ER doctors in the Arlington area, recruiting many excellent residency-trained ER doctors, added our own scribes and PAs to keep up with the changing times in Emergency Medicine. Arlington Emergency Medical Associates was the only formal ER residency trained group to have ever staffed that hospital until June of 2017, which is when my life was turned upside down and we were taken over by Emergency Medical Care, Inc. in an "alleged" merger. It was forced upon us and all attempts to hold the contract failed.

During my stay at AMH, I became chief of staff, was on the AMH Board and Medical Executive Committee for many years. Arlington Emergency Medical Associates added another hospital to their contracts which I negotiated, and that was USMD Hospital at Arlington, which we had for eight years. Times were changing and it's true nothing stays the same. An interesting note is that Emergency Medical Consultants (EMC) announced in December of 2017, only after six months at AMH, they were in the process of selling out to a nationwide ER group: Team Health. They had been negotiating for six months on this merger.

I've learned never to trust administrators or health systems. They will do what they want. They say they want to partner with doctors, but that's BS. Unless you're big money to them they don't care. Neurosurgical, orthopedics, and cardiovascular bring in big money to these healthcare systems. The market shareholders and administration bend over backward for these doctors. But ER doctors? Big money could care less. I always looked at the ER as my practice, but we really never had total control over the overall operations.

Many things have changed in EM. Once you would

have never gotten a CT scan for a suspected appendix. A diagnosis was based on history, exam, and lab data. Nowadays, the surgeons want CTs on everything. Ultrasound uses in the ER and ultrasound-guided central lines have become the standard. One day, when I placed a central line blindly, these new young doctors were amazed I did not use ultrasound.

Times, they were a changing.

Chapter 26
Introduction to Adrian Cheong, MD

Dr. Cheong joined our group soon after its inception in 1990. Early on, it became obvious to me that he had an exceptional knowledge of emergency medicine, and that opinion never wavered. He seemed to be a "go to" guy for complicated cases, and very thoughtfully and meticulously cared for his patients. He, along with several other partners, helped to make our ER exceptional and me a better emergency doctor.

Dr. Cheong came into the world in Port of Spain, Republic of Trinidad & Tobago on January 7, 1944, the oldest of four children. He received the highest marks and won the mathematics prize in Port of Spain while in 12th grade.

Chapter 27
Dr. Adrian Cheong's Story

The Knife

2:14 a.m.

A nurse called out to me. “Hey, Dr. Cheong, I have a patient in bed #2 of the ward. He complains of back pain and doesn't appear to be in any distress,” the nurse reported on the patient that had just checked in. The department was almost empty.

I greeted a 40-something-year-old, well-built male patient with sandy brown hair, seated comfortably on the gurney. I listened to his complaint of chronic low back pain, which apparently worsened that night. Other than the smell of alcohol and mild tenderness in the lower back, the exam was normal. We discussed my diagnosis and management plan with him, including a prescription for an NSAID.

He wanted an opiate. “NSAIDs just don’t work.” I explained my rationale for his treatment, including the use of NSAIDs, which was based on his clinical exam.

This wasn't acceptable to him. He said that he wasn't appreciated for all that he has done “for you and for you f*****g hongs in Vietnam!”

I excused myself and walked into the nurse’s lounge, where both of my nurses sat. I stood in the doorway and explained that security needed to be called because the patient became upset and belligerent. I looked at Linda, one of my nurses, and her expression changed to one of fear. She blinked, looking upwards, then at me in the doorway. I immediately turned around. The patient filled the space behind me. I walked into the room and he quickly followed, producing a knife with a huge blade. All three of us faced him. Me standing. My two nurses sitting. Linda spoke in a soothing voice, trying to get him back to his room. He didn't appear to hear her. He continued his belligerence with the use of expletives. She reassured him that this could be resolved amicably. He still didn't seem to hear. He continued to stand in the doorway, waving this huge knife, mumbling about his Vietnam days and all the "f*****g hongs" that he had saved, while almost being killed.

Susan, the other nurse, sat quietly, her left hand on the phone. Unfortunately, there was only one way in and out of the room and that's where the patient stood. He approached. We stood our ground. Linda continued to talk about getting this resolved in his room. He cursed and swore.

I looked around the small room—not a lot in there except a few chairs and a table. There were three of us against this one individual. If only we could summon security without alarming him. In the event that he lunged and needed to be disarmed, I thought I would go for his knife. I would grab his right arm and wrestle it out of his hand. The other two would restrain him.

Instead, we collectively thanked him for his service and what he had done for us all. He retreated and mumbled. Then, he turned and started walking out of the room. Susan called security. The patient walked through the department and subsequently left. Security finally arrived but the immediate crisis was over. They I scoured the campus to make sure that he had left.

Becoming a doctor, continuing the grueling practice, reminds me of my racing days. Consider this memory:

The Race
By Adrian Cheong, MD

Drenched in sweat, like I just stepped out of the shower (That might be an over-exaggeration, maybe not that wet.), I looked ahead. My brother, Stephen, beckoned to me, "Come on up, boy, come up here." I stayed right where I was, in the middle of the pack, and to the left side of this mass of humanity.

December in Barbados is hot, humid, and steamy, the third annual Independence Day Run. I had just arrived from Antigua the day before to join my brother and other members of the Road Runners Club of Trinidad and Tobago.

I had spent a week in St. Kitts at a small, locally-owned resort tucked away on the side of a mountain, a quaint little place owned by a friend of my grandparents, Mrs. Lamb. Amid the lush tropical greenery, the mango and orange trees, the banana plants, and anthurium lilies stood five or six wooden cabins.

During my stay, I had done one 10K run and that was from the resort to Basse Terre, the capital. I had needed a comb, so decided to run into the city to get one. It was a straight shot. I headed left as I departed the resort, then followed the main road into town. It was a hot, miserable endeavor in the middle of the day; the shoulder of the road at times consisted of gravel and I could feel the cars as they whizzed by. I was the object of stares from foreign students attending Ross

University, an offshore medical school, and occasional toots from taxis. Strangely enough, no one stopped to offer me a ride. Maybe it was because I was too sweaty. Who knows?

Eventually, I ended up at the pharmacy. I presented a sweat-drenched five dollar bill, which the pharmacist had to dry off. He stared at me, soaking wet, and commented on it being a nice day.

Running, or more accurately jogging, back to the resort was less tedious, but with the same road hazards - cars whizzing by in close proximity and the need to watch my footing on the gravel shoulder. That was the extent of my training for the event in Barbados.

The mild breeze from the ocean didn't give much relief from the heat generated by some one thousand runners all bunched up at the starting line. I saw Stephen, Saloum, Sam, Pecos, Gregory, and Gary up front. I liked the middle of the pack. I could pass a few runners and not be on the heels of the faster runners. Being on the outside, I could, if necessary, do some overtaking by using the sidewalk. I looked around. There were all shapes, sizes, and colors of runners, mostly young and black. There were a few white faces. The start was at the upper end of the local race track where, on my left, I saw a hint of the blue Caribbean Sea. With each moment that passed, my anxiety increased. *How will the race go? What will my time be? Am I going to achieve a Personal Record (PR) here?*

The wait drove me nuts. Everyone else appeared as anxious and ready to get this race moving as I was. Loud static over the PA startled me back to the ready. Officials welcomed us to the island and thanked us for making it another successful event. The crowd roared. I glanced ahead. My brother called to me again to join the group up front. I stayed put. The start shot split the air. We started moving. I walked to the start line. It took a minute-and-a-half to get there. I continued walking after I passed the first kilometer. It was too crowded. I had to get moving. Finding a path amid a few runners, I wove through, now jogging. I looked ahead and couldn't see the rest of my team.

Down the streets lined with spectators, I tried to find my stride. We were heading into Bridgetown, the capital. I couldn’t focus on the sights around me, I stayed on pace.

The crowds continued to cheer. I could tell by my breathing that I had found my stride. I heard a continuous flip-flop sound that seemed to be keeping stride with me—right behind me, then alongside me. I tried to focus on what was ahead of me and not glance to my left. I focused on the road, avoiding the camber and potholes.

The crowds lining the course in Bridgetown appeared to be cheering and focusing on me. Bewildered, not only by the flip-flopping alongside me but by the attention I seemed to be receiving. I accelerated and so did the pitter-patter. I couldn't seem to shake this person. It was most annoying and I was pissed.

I glanced to the left through the corner of my eye to see what was there. It was this kid, maybe eleven years old, who was striding alongside me, with no shoes on. I couldn't believe it. He was running barefoot.

I couldn't let this youngster kick my ass – no sir! I looked around. We were still downtown. The buildings cast a shadow on the street. The pack was thinning out. There was more room for acceleration. The Trini team –

my brother, Pecos, Saloum, Sam, and Gregory were nowhere to be seen. They had to be way ahead. As I started passing other runners, my breathing became rapid and deep.

A blond-headed runner dashed from the course into the crowd. I didn't know what that was all about. I had to stay focused on ending the race in a good time. The course turned from downtown into what appeared to be a residential area, with homes right up to the curb of the very narrow streets. There were no sidewalks.

There was no traffic and now I could just see a few runners ahead of me. I was suffering. My glasses were slipping off my sweaty face. Sweat poured off my arms, beads of sweat dripped from my hands. I hurt, feeling as if I was going to die on this course. *Where is the end to this pain and suffering? I can't stop now.*

On this stretch there were no crowds lining the street. It was desolate. I looked ahead and about two kilometers away, I saw the back of a tall, thin runner. It looked like Gregory. I tried to catch up to him but he suddenly spurted ahead in a burst of energy. I couldn't keep up. *I'm going to die right here. Where is the end to this misery? God, I hope it's just around the next corner.*

It wasn't. I closed my eyes for a few minutes to wipe the sweat out of them – which didn't work because my sweaty fingers wiped more sweat into them. This was the worst I had ever felt in a race. My stomach cramped. Nauseated, I felt I would vomit. Lo and behold, I turned into a street that led to the park—the end of the race. Stephen, my brother, stood about one kilometer from the finish line, cheering me on, pushing me harder.

"Go, Cheongie, go, go, go!"

I crossed the finish-line and looked at the clock—

thirty-six minutes and some seconds. My knees wobbled. I asked for water. Gasping, I took a sip. It made me more nauseated. I needed to sit. I needed to lie down. Finally, a spot in the grass blurred before me and I laid down. *Made it!* My first international race – unofficially representing Trinidad and Tobago – ended.

Chapter 28
God and the Doctor

Retirement has given me time for all the things I couldn't do in my working years. There's time for things like making my very first girlfriend my wife and best friend, fishing in Alaska or writing a book. I have time to read something other than medical journals. One thing I had always wanted to read was the Bible.

It must have been sometime in the 1940s when I first thought about my beliefs. The preacher said, "Son, do you love Jesus? Do you accept Jesus as your Lord and Savior?" I knew the right answer, but did I really love Jesus? I didn't know Jesus. I knew my mother, my father, my sister, and brother, and I loved them, but I didn't know Jesus. This breach of godliness scared me. I didn't want to go to hell, as the preacher said I would if I didn't believe, but it is also a sin to lie, and if I said yes, *I love Jesus*, it felt like a lie.

Do normal kids really love Jesus and God, or do they just claim to do so to please their parents and the preacher? Is it right to baptize a child and ask those serious questions of one who doesn't actually know what he or she is admitting to? This is standard procedure in many religions, but not all. Christening doesn't require a response from an infant or small child. This treatise refers to those who do require such response.

My personal dilemma concerned me for most of my early life and was aggravated by my ignorance of Christianity. My lack of knowledge finally gave me an excuse to almost totally ignore religion for many years, but I still found myself praying at times of unusual adversity, for my family, myself. and later for my patients. I thanked God for His help on those occasions.

My college years found me in a state of poverty. Hunger became a frequent part of my existence. My general deficiencies of the necessities of life depressed me. There didn't appear to be real hope of improvement in the foreseeable future. I flunked out of college. Lack of money meant I couldn't have continued anyway. I might have prayed for help then, but I don't remember doing so.

I got a job, but then West Texas oil fields suffered a downturn in the early 1950s, and jobs for unskilled people like me were scarce. Perhaps, unknown to me, providence apparently came to my rescue when my brother secured a job for me and allowed me to live with him and his family. During the months of work and relative solitude, I made the decision to work toward a degree in biology with the hope of entering medical school. By the spring semester, my old nemesis, hunger, returned to haunt me, but my resolve to continue was unshaken. I wondered, was I being tested in more ways than academics? My medical practice dominated my time and became my mistress, much to the detriment of my personal life, as two divorces will attest.

When I thought about spiritual things, I hoped that my dedication to the welfare and healing of my patients was enough to bring salvation, but I remained ignorant of Christianity. At the ripe age of 80 years, I accomplished a lifelong desire to read the Bible. I had tried on occasion, but failed. Now, with the encouragement of my new wife, Zotyne, I accomplished the reading, then I felt compelled to join the church. I had never felt comfortable in a church, nor had I known a pastor who impressed me greatly until a friend and high school teammate, Ralph Turner, introduced me to the Church on Thistle Ridge in Granbury, Texas. I immediately connected with Pastor C.C. Risenhoover and his beliefs on life and Christianity. The church has become important to me, and I'm learning about faith. I'm now capable of understanding the meaning of the word and The Word. My wife saw in me a need unfulfilled, and her impetus spurred me on. I am grateful. I have been baptized, testifying to the statement, I do love Jesus.

Chapter 29
Regret, Hope, and Heroes

A Note of Regret:

I would have enjoyed stories from more of my partners, but, for various reasons, several of those I did contact were unable to contribute to the book and some I couldn't locate.

My Hope:

I hope that by sharing these stories I painted a picture of the history of Emergency Medicine, a profile of the work of emergency physicians and the heart of the doctors who serve—the Heroes who save lives.

DOCTORS WORKING IN THE AMH AREA ER:

A LIST OF ER DOCTORS - 1970 TO 1990

Bohn Allen, Kent Cherry, Frank Flory, Gaston Machado, Darwin Hale, Thomas Lavake, Doyle Lansford, Gerald Thompson, Barna Richards, Donna Baker, Gilbert Ledesma, George Anagnostis, William Bowers, Frank DelaTorre. If I forgot someone, forgive me. It has been a long time.

A List of ER Doctors at AMH - 1990 to 2007

Richard Neville, Mary Rae, Jane Torgerson, Debbie Lund, Adrian Cheong, Roy Yamada, Barna Richards,

Frank Flory, Andrea Green, Danny Kocurek, Hoyt Frenzel, Brad Kipp, Alex Geslani, Jon Beesley, Larry Gayao, Travis Coates, Yama Amin, Larry Chien, Joseph Delprincipe, Howell Davis, and Matt Way.

To the Barna Richards
A NOTE OF RECOGNITION
From Staff and Patient at Time of Retirement

Dear Dr. Richards,

Thank you for the hard work, dedication and sacrifices that you have made over the years at Arlington Memorial Hospital. Under your leadership, the "Emergency Room" has literally been built into a full-service "Emergency Department" that cares for nearly 70,000 patients per year.

We are the safety net for the citizens of Arlington and Tarrant County—open twenty-four hours a day, seven days a week; on weekends and holidays; during times of sleet or snow; and seeing everyone, regardless of their ability to pay.

You should be very proud of what you have created. The seed that you planted many years ago will continue to nurtured and cultivated. It will continue to grow. It will serve many patients in the years to come. Your legacy will continue to live on.

With the deepest appreciation,
Your Staff and Patients

About The Author
Barna A. Richards, M. D., FACEP

Born in 1935, in Weatherford, Texas, Barna Richards grew up in Ranger and Wink, Texas. He attended Wink High School, played on the 1952 state championship football team and graduated in 1954. His career began at North Texas State College (now UNT) in pre-med and he graduated in 1959 with a BA in biology.

Dr. Richards received his MD at the University of Texas Medical Branch, Galveston, Texas, where he attended medical school from 1959 until 1963.

Internship and family practice residency: John Peter Smith Hospital Fort Worth, Texas - 1963 until 1965.

Private practice, solo practice, family medicine - 1965 to 1991. He worked in the ER during these years, nights and weekends.

Medical Director and staff physician of, emergency department Arlington Memorial Hospital - 1987 to 2006

Medical Director, EMS, City of Arlington, Texas - 1987 to 1997.

Medical Director, EMS, City of Pantego - 1988 to 1996, monitored and taught cardiac and trauma care to paramedics.

Board certified in emergency medicine - 1988 re-certified in 1998.

Affiliate Faculty, American Heart Association, for Advanced Cardiac Life Support - 1991 to 2002.

Taught and monitored courses on ACLS to students, nurses, paramedics, and physicians.

Hospital Affiliations:

Arlington Memorial Hospital medical staff - 1965 to 2008, Chairman and member of various committees.

Medical Director, Emergency Department - 1986 to 2006.

HCA (now Columbia HCA) - 1965 to approximately 1985, resigned due to excess time required for two hospital commitments.

Millwood Hospital, Arlington, Texas, medical clearance for admitted patients, March, 2012. Resigned, didn't like it.

Designated doctor for Texas Worker's Compensation Commission for impairment ratings for injured workers until retired in 2015.

Currently does medical disability exams for Social Security Disability.

Certified by the National Registration of Certified Medical Examiners to examine truck drivers with commercial licenses. Certification #: 2796093983

Worked part-time for Concentra Medical Clinics in occupational medicine and urgent care from 2006 to February, 2015. These clinics are located in the DFW metroplex: Dallas, Fort Worth, Arlington, Burleson, Carrollton, Addison, Las Colinas, Garland, and Mesquite, working one to three shifts per week and treating 20 to 30 patients, occasionally more, per nine-hour shift.

Retired from Concentra in February, 2015.

Community Activities:

Physician for well-baby clinic, exams and immunizations for indigent infants and young children, ten years - 1965 to 1975

Physician for pediatric clinic for indigent children, ten years - 1965 to 1975

Team physician for Lamar High School, Arlington, Texas - 1970 to 1991

Board of directors, Arlington Boys Club, two terms

Physician for Home for Aged Masons, ten years

Physical exams for Boys Club sports, ten years - 1965 to 1975

Physical exams and monitor for UTA intramural boxing tournaments, various years

Physician for UTA handicapped students - 1975 to 1985

Physical exams for Pee Wee Football, several years

Teaching:

ACLS (Advanced Cardiac Life Support) for paramedics, physicians, and nurses, twenty years

BTLS (trauma protocols) for paramedics, ten years

Taught various emergency topics to nurses and paramedics

Taught prep courses to Texas Emergency Physicians for board preparation

Gave lectures on various topics to city employees

Monitored students in office for Health Occupations classes

Research Activities:

- Various studies on parasitology in medical school; did in vitro research in dogs on Methicillin
- Studies on various pain relievers, antibiotics, and anti-depressants for Sandoz Pharmaceutical, twenty-two years
- Pre-release clinical studies on Imitrex, a migraine drug, for Glaxo Pharmaceutical

Never sanctioned by a hospital, the medical society, or the Texas State Board of Medical Examiners.

Became certified to perform exams for the VA on injured military personnel applying for service-connected benefits in 2012.

Chosen “Physician of the Year” by the Arlington Medical Association Medical Society, December, 2007.

To contact Dr. Barna Richards email:
Barna.Richards@yahoo.com

Made in the USA
Las Vegas, NV
26 December 2020

14751393R00095